GETTING H[illegible]Y NATURALLY

JOHN BYRNE N.D., B.H.Sc.

Ireland's Foremost Naturopath

First Published in Ireland, in 2015, in co-operation with Choice Publishing,

Drogheda, County Louth, Republic of Ireland.

www.choicepublishing.ie

ISBN: 978-1-909154-79-7

About the Author

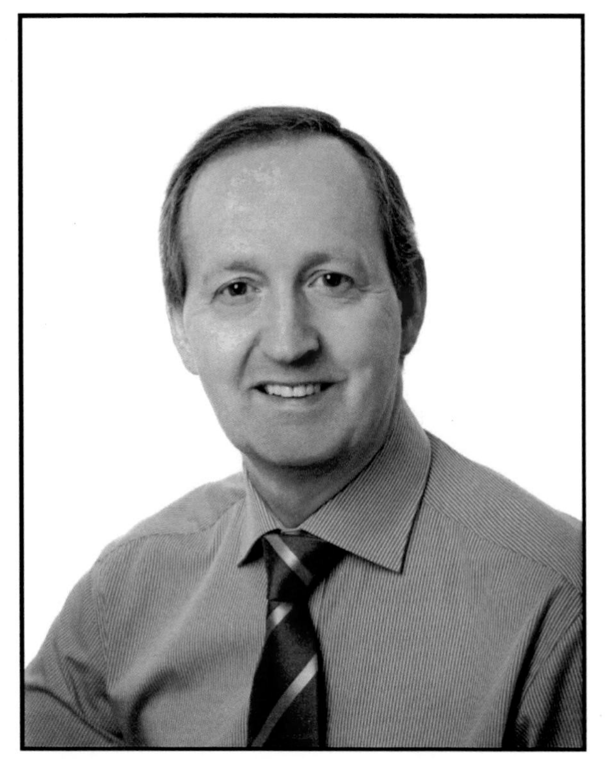

John Byrne N.D., B.H.Sc. is a naturopathic physician having received his training in Australia, where he obtained a Bachelor of Health Science from the University of New England, along with an Advanced Diploma in Naturopathy from Nature Care College in Sydney, as well as Diplomas in Herbal Medicine, Nutrition, Remedial Massage and Lymphatic Drainage Massage.

John has been involved in natural healing therapies since 1990 and it is his fervent belief that most health problems are reversible. He currently lives in Navan, Co. Meath where he has been running a busy natural healing practice for the past fifteen years.

Due to the diverse and eclectic nature of his studies and his many years experience as a practicing naturopath and nutritional consultant, John understands that vibrant health can only evolve through a process that involves the integration of body, mind and spirit. In his healing work with individuals, he develops health plans based on dietary and lifestyle practices to create a new vision of health and vitality.

If you have benefited from information in this book or would like to consult further with John regarding appointments then please phone his clinic at 046-9060702 and check his website at: www.naturaltherapy.ie

Dedicated

This book is dedicated to you – the promoter of your own health, and also, to those humans among us, who suffer needlessly – unaware that simple, safe and effective ways of correcting their ailments and restoring themselves to health are available.

Acknowledgements

I wish to thank my wife Beulah – my ever loving and supportive companion, without whose love, help and encouragement this book would never have reached completion.

To my two young children Shane and Olivia – who lost their dad to his computer most evenings and weekends, month after month – such patience and love! They mean the world to me.

And to my clients throughout the years – It's been an honour and privilege to be a part of your care.

John Byrne N.D., B.H.Sc.

TABLE OF CONTENTS

INTRODUCTION

When it comes to our health we know instinctively that people who pay attention to health and wellness measures in their lifestyle enjoy better health and longevity compared to those who are less rigorous about optimal lifestyle habits. These days there is undoubtedly a greater public awareness of what constitutes healthy lifestyle factors (i.e. sensible diet, pure water, clean air, exercise, emotional harmony, adequate sleep, etc). However, our fast-paced modern lifestyles have taken us off the right track with fast foods, excessive alcohol consumption, smoking and other drug dependencies, a polluted environment and high stress levels. These unhealthy lifestyle habits, which have developed over many years, can be very difficult to change. And so rather than making the effort to take the necessary steps well in advance of a health problem occurring we, like the proverbial ostrich who sticks its head in the sand tend to ignore our health status until obvious illness strikes.

Here's a question: Have you ever wondered how sick you actually are at this moment in time? Think about it, it's a tough one to answer. You certainly know when you have back pain, suffer the odd headache or experience seasonal allergies. But are you otherwise healthy? Do you simply view good health as the absence of pain, illness or disease? To help you with these questions, consider The World Health Organisation's definition of health as **"not merely the absence of disease, but instead, a vibrant state of wellbeing and enjoyment of life!"** In 1946 the World Health Organisation (WHO) defined health as: "A state of complete physical, mental and social wellbeing, not just the absence of disease or infirmity".

Judging by the above holistic definition of health, not suffering from any apparent ailments does not necessarily mean that you have a rosy future. Outward appearance and lack of physical illness markers are not reliable barometers of health. Even thin people can have hypertension, high cholesterol, fatty livers, diabetes and heart disease.

Or maybe you're of the belief that your health status is predetermined at birth by the genetic markers that predispose you to certain serious health ailments. If you are genetically marked for cancer, you will likely get cancer. If you are genetically destined for diabetes or Parkinson's disease, you can only do your best to slow down their onset by making good diet and lifestyle choices and hope for the best. This mythical belief that genetics dictate our disease risk, one that has been fostered upon us by the medical establishment may at first sound plausible, but a new emerging field of Epigenetics tears to shreds this old paradigm of genetics being the cause of most health conditions.(1)

Still it seems most people are happy to continue believing this myth. It's easier to blame heredity than it is to take responsibility for your own health. Heart disease is not your fault; it "runs in your family". You're not responsible for your diabetes; sure, didn't your mother and your aunt both have it! You must have inherited a genetic weakness. And it can't be your fault that you're fat, after all, just

Epigenetics

Epigenetics is the study of changes in gene expression, in other words how genes are turned on and off. There are 25,000 genes in your DNA and the scientific premise that these genes control your life has one major flaw: genes cannot turn themselves on and off, they are just blueprints. Instead, something in the environment has to trigger gene activity.

The term epigenetics, meaning "control above genetics", is a new science of how environmental and lifestyle factors can select genes and modify the readout of these genes for better or for worse. In other words, what you eat and drink, whether your smoke, take recreational drugs or medications, what environmental pollutants you encounter and even what beliefs, emotions and attitudes you hold, can all affect gene expression.

This is significant because we can become masters of our genes and their expression because we can actually control our health by our choice of dietary and lifestyle factors including our psychological health.

about everybody in your family is overweight. You must have the same "slow metabolism"!

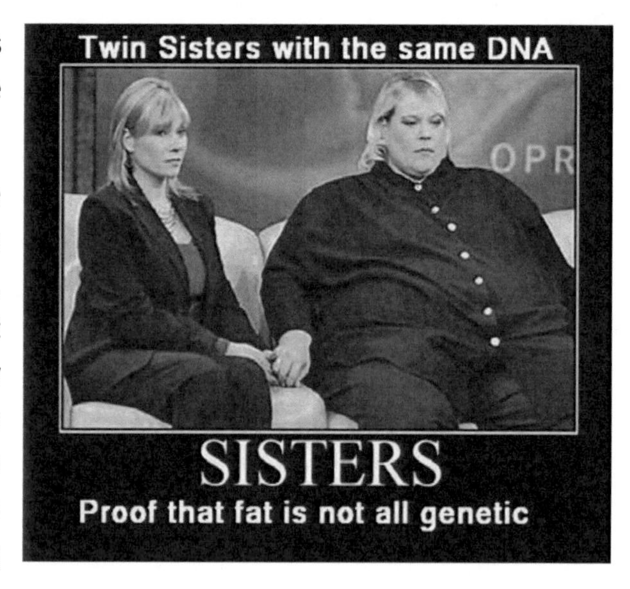

People who think this way are much more likely to pop a pill when something goes wrong. After all, what's the use in trying to prevent something if you're already destined for it? These people are also more likely to seek the assistance of doctors rather than focus on prevention and taking responsibility for their own health.

However, in the vast majority of cases, it is not our genetics that puts us at risk of health conditions such as obesity, diabetes, heart disease or cancer. It is our poor dietary habits and lifestyle choices. The only reason why heart disease "runs in the family" is because the same "disease-causing habits" run in the family.

Craig Venter, one of the leading scientists behind the sequencing of the human genetic code had this to say about the role of genetics as it relates to our risk for disease: *"Human biology is far more complicated that we imagine. Everybody talks about genes that they received from their mother and father, for this trait or the other. But in reality, those genes have very little impact on the outcomes. Our biology is far too complicated for that and deals with hundreds of thousands of independent factors. Genes are absolutely not our fate".*

Instead, our modern diet and lifestyle are the main culprits for the explosion of chronic degenerative diseases occurring in our society today. The shame of it is that they are largely preventable. Although diet is only one of many important lifestyle factors implicated in the cause of this group of diseases, countless studies have shown that eating a healthy and adequate diet provides a significant protective role against the development of chronic disease.

Eating a healthy diet also increases our general wellbeing. How many of us on a daily basis complain of things like tiredness and not feeling a hundred percent even when there is nothing drastically wrong? If you settle for what seems to be average health, then you are not as healthy as you could be. Choosing to make positive changes to your diet and lifestyle choices can quickly improve your health status making your life immeasurably better.

Eating the right amounts of the right types of food as well as incorporating other health promoting practices such as regular exercise, stress management, rest and adequate sleep, and avoiding smoking and excessive alcohol consumption can mean the difference between dragging yourself through each day and truly living and getting the most out of life while also preventing the development of any serious disease.

My focus on health through the years from a naturopathic perspective maintains that one's primary goal should be 'health creation' rather than 'disease eradication' and that most efforts towards health creation should be self-directed using the building blocks of nature such as a sensible diet, pure water, sunshine, fresh air, regular exercise as well as cultivating a positive mental attitude.

If you think about it, the human body is an amazing system that is designed to strive towards health, not disease. Disease is simply a defensive reaction by the body to poor dietary and lifestyle habits. The symptoms of disease are the remedial efforts of the body attempting a cleansing process in an effort to rid itself of accumulated toxins. As such, the power to cure disease resides only within the patient's body and that innate healing power cannot fully prevail until wrong living habits stop and the fundamental elements of nature in fitting measure, have been set in place. Properly managed, the disease process is also the road to cure.

Wouldn't it be nice then if one could quickly hone in on exactly what needs to be rectified when the body is struck down by illness? New research findings show that most diseases of affluence have simple explanations and cures once their true cause is known. So what if I told you that all the major health conditions plaguing mankind today share a common underlying trait that more and more researchers now believe to be the ultimate cause of ill health!

There is now a growing mountain of evidence in the medical literature of a shared symptom, a common trait, underlying all chronic degenerative conditions. This common denominator is INFLAMMATION, or more technically 'low-grade chronic inflammation' or 'systemic inflammation'.

Over recent years the role of inflammation as a causative factor in the etiology of many disease conditions has become a huge area of interest in the medical world. There has literally been an explosion of information coming out of the medical literature linking inflammation with a myriad of health conditions. It's associated with nearly every modern disease including many dreaded diseases such as: heart disease, diabetes, multiple sclerosis, cancer, Alzheimer's, dementia, Parkinson's, any condition that ends in "itis", e.g. arthritis, as well as insidious conditions like obesity, fibromyalgia, chronic fatigue, depression and so on.

Wouldn't it be nice then if one could learn how to eliminate this inflammation from the body, thereby rendering oneself practically free of developing any chronic disease later in life........

READ ON....

CHAPTER 1

HEALTH – WHERE TO START

> *"Let your food be your medicine, and*
> *Your medicine be your food" - Hippocrates*

We all try, we really do! We believe in the value of a good diet so we try to eat well. We remember the admonition of our parents to eat a good breakfast; we know it to be the most important meal of the day.

We do the best we can, we try to eat regularly, choose foods carefully and cut back on what we know is wrong. When we think of it, we order a salad instead of a burger and chips; and we try to eat our vegetables.

We try not to skip meals unless it's absolutely necessary. We know that too many sweets are bad for us, so we deny ourselves most of the time and we don't order dessert at every meal.

But we get busy.....appointments, deadlines, schedules, children, school runs, the list never ends! And so, in our busy lifestyle, it is difficult to be that disciplined with our eating habits. The way we live is often a race with the clock and so, fast foods or pre-prepared meals can be easier to fit into our busy lifestyle equation.

Our society has made it easier for us to eat out or grab a take-away and more difficult because of the time involved to prepare meals at home. Just take a look at your own town or locality; it seems like every other street corner has a fast food outlet of some kind!

And besides...... we don't do it that often and our health does not appear to be suffering too much; a few extra kilos here and there maybe, but nothing too serious! Sure! Isn't our life expectancy getting longer and longer, so how can modern convenience foods cause any major health issues?

But are we really doing OK? Take into consideration our overstretched healthcare system that's unable to cope with the hugely increased demand for its services as a result of epidemic proportions of degenerative diseases affecting people today. Over fifty years of medical research has conclusively shown that most common diseases today are related at least in part to diet. This is particularly true in the case of heart disease and many cancers, which are the two major causes of death in the developed World at present and are on an ever-increasing scale.(2)

Over those past fifty years medical and scientific research has revealed that saturated fats, white flour, refined carbohydrates, high red meat consumption along with the increasing amount of chemical additives and pesticide laden foods, are all major contributors to the development of poor health and disease states. Indeed, the medical establishment now acknowledge the central role diet plays in a person's overall health status.

'When diet is wrong, medicine is of no use. When diet is correct, medicine is of no need."

~ Ancient Ayurvedic Proverb

Your daily dietary choices can influence your risk of developing an imposing list of life-shortening diseases including diabetes, stroke, heart disease, cancer, auto-immune diseases, Alzheimer's, arthritis, not to mention the less threatening conditions such as obesity, osteoporosis or even tooth decay.

Many of us, even those who feel they eat well, do not eat a nutritionally balanced diet. We tend to eat too much of the wrong sorts of fats (hydrogenated, saturated and an imbalance of omega-3 to omega-6 fats), far too much sugar; too much animal protein and an excess calorie intake. A great deal of the calories we consume on a daily basis come from highly processed convenience or snack foods that are rich in fat and sugar.

A famous study carried out by the U.S. government in the 1970's originally called the HANES study, now referred to as: NHANES 1 (National Health and Nutrition Examination Survey), found that the general population really didn't know much about nutrition or how to choose a healthy diet, or if they did know, they choose not to apply their knowledge. The result of the NHANES 1 study was of such concern to the U.S. policy makers that a ten year effort was embarked upon to improve people's awareness of the importance of good nutrition. The hope was that by getting people to improve their diets, one would see a reduction in the incidence of diet-related diseases. Following ten years of effort, the same survey was again conducted on the U.S. population and called NHANES II. The results were disappointing to say the least; the problem had actually gotten worse! (3)

Although this was an American study, if we consider the increased incidence of diet-related diseases in Ireland today, compared to in the past when people mostly ate at home, then we can easily extrapolate from the NHANES study, that were a similar study ever to be carried out here, we would in all probability get similar results, meaning that the average Irish diet of today is not that healthy.

So where are we going wrong? In our society the vast majority of us are lucky enough to be able to meet our basic needs of food and accommodation. There is no need or reason as to why we can't eat well; and often a healthy diet is cheaper than a highly refined and overly processed diet. More often than not, our food choices seem to be based on what tastes good and not necessarily what is good for us. Paradoxically, it is possible to eat good healthy nutritious food that actually tastes good. And because of the improved state of health often experienced when we change our eating patterns, the unhealthy foods we previously craved generally become less attractive.

Another factor that influences our food choices is time restrictions. The way we live is often a race with the clock and so fast foods or pre-prepared meals can be easier to fit into our lifestyle equation. This is where priority comes in - diet is the cornerstone of health and should be given the focus and attention it deserves. The interesting thing is that healthy food often comes ready to go, and simple easy-to-make meals can be prepared in short amounts of time with only a small amount of organization. More and more food outlets are now providing a menu selection that provides the opportunity for good food choices.

So let's take a look at what makes up a healthy diet and how this type of diet can taste good as well as being good for you.

The Basics of Good Nutrition:

A healthy diet may be defined as one which meets the body's requirement for energy and essential nutrients without providing excess; that are obtained from a variety of foods and that minimize the risks for diet-related diseases.(4)

Research suggests that diets which best meet the requirement of "healthful diets" are based on the consumption of a variety of whole foods, staying as close to nature as possible by eating lots of fresh fruits, vegetables, grains, nuts, beans and seeds, with lean meats, chicken, fish and dairy products as accompaniments. Such diets tend to be high in plant foods, complex carbohydrates, vitamins and minerals, and low in saturated fats, salt and calories.

A basic diet needs to provide at a minimum, adequate calories from carbohydrates, protein and fat along with vitamins and minerals necessary to metabolize those calories. Unfortunately a high percentage of our daily food intake tends to be made up of "empty calorie" foods. These are foods high in calories but low in the vitamins and minerals required to metabolize those calories. We call them "junk foods".

These empty calorie foods do not provide sufficient vitamins and minerals and therefore they rob these micronutrients from the rest of the diet and also from our body tissues in order to metabolize the calories found in such foods. These junk foods should be eliminated or at least kept to a minimum.

The first step then to achieving optimal health is to start paying closer attention to your diet. We are now all pretty familiar with the "food pyramid". The lower levels of this pyramid, which should also make up the base of a good diet is high in fruits, vegetables and grains. The top of the pyramid represents the foods that should be reduced in the diet or eliminated altogether and include "junk food" already discussed as empty calorie foods.

Variety:

Variety in the diet is essential if you want to obtain the proper balance of needed nutrients and to avoid possible excesses of toxic substances. Besides, a varied diet is more interesting than an unvaried one. There are many highly nutritious foods such as fruits, grains, beans, nuts and varieties of vegetables that few of us currently eat. And there are dozens of tasty new ways to combine familiar ingredients that you may never have thought of before. Try looking at some cookbooks written to promote healthier eating, you may be pleasantly surprised. Experimentation with culinary herbs and different flavour combinations can also be fun.

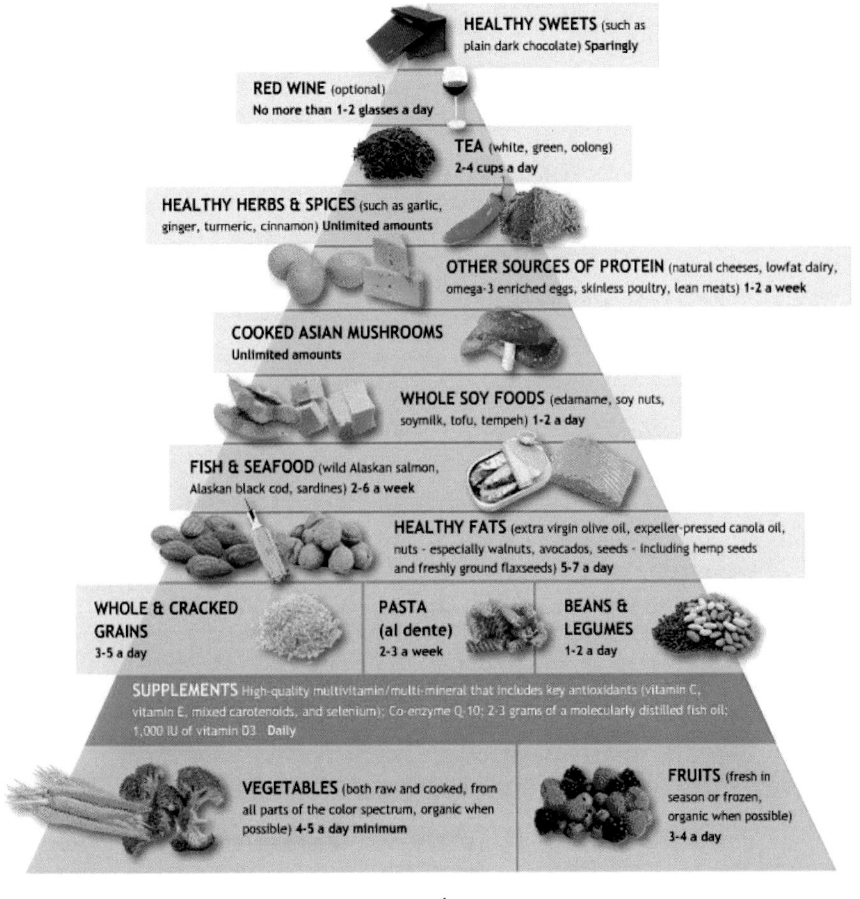

Moderation:

Healthy nutrition is not an all-or-nothing phenomenon, but a matter of putting more emphasis on some foods and less on others. Unless you have a health problem that requires you to steer clear of certain foods, there's no reason why you need to give up any food you especially like. A dish of ice-cream for dessert every night is not healthy, (too much fat and sugar and too many calories) but there's nothing wrong with ice-cream once a week.

Moderation also means portion control. If you eat a large steak at one meal, you'll be taking in too much fat and cholesterol and too many calories to meet your dietary guidelines. But if your serving is a small portion of steak, you can stay within the guidelines. Remember, you need a lot less food for good health than you may think.

EAT ALL THE COLOURS OF THE RAINBOW

RED: raspberries, strawberries, goji berries, cranberries, water melon, apples, tomatoes, peppers, radishes, rhubarb.
ORANGE: oranges, mango, apricots, honeydew melon, walnuts, sweet potatoes, pumpkins, turnips, butternut squash, carrots.
YELLOW: bananas, lemons, pears, grapefruit, honey, pineapple, corn, eggs, chickpeas, quinoa, ginger, turmeric, olive oil, millet.
GREEN: cabbage, broccoli, brussel sprouts, spinach, kale, asparagus, celery, peas, peppers, avocado, apples, kiwi fruit, gooseberries.
BLUE: blueberries, blue grapes.
PURPLE: plums, purple grapes, boysenberries, elderberries, cherries, blackcurrants, red cabbage, beetroot, eggplant, red onions.
WHITE: coconuts, potatoes, cauliflower, parsnips, white beans, onions, garlic, oats, mushrooms.

More Nutritional Hot Tips:

Reduce simple sugars from your diet. Simple sugars such as table sugar, soft drinks, lollies and sweets have little nutritional value. It is said that the average person consumed between one and two kilograms of sugar per year in the early 1900's. Today a person consumes more than their body weight of sugar per year. Sugar provides no vitamins or minerals to the body but uses up much of our existing vitamin B supplies for its own catabolism. The B vitamins are extremely important to health and particularly for the nervous system. About 98% of chromium present in sugarcane is lost in turning it into sugar.(5) Chromium is vital for keeping blood sugar levels stable. (Note: blackstrap molasses, a natural derivative of sugar cane is rich in chromium and many other minerals and is a good food supplement. Take a dessertspoonful daily).

White (bleached) flour used in many confectionary products, offers no nutrition and is harmful to the body. Rather, use unrefined flours made from rice, millet, rye, barley, corn, soy and buckwheat.

Avoid as much as possible hydrogenated fats and oils commonly used in fried foods, especially in deep fried takeaways where oil has been reheated many times. Reheating oil can produce carcinogenic substances.

Use cold pressed oils such as olive and coconut oil for cooking, linseed, sunflower and safflower oils for dressings. Also include in your diet a variety of nuts, seeds, avocados, oily fish, supplements such as cod liver oil, evening primrose oil and omega-3 fish oils. These foods are rich in omega-3 & 6 essential fatty acids that are very important to the body especially for the nervous system, the heart and circulation, the skin and the hormonal and glandular system. Every cell has a membrane which is partly lipid (fat), therefore dietary fats from healthy sources help to keep each and every cell healthy and functioning well. A fatty sheath (the myelin sheath) provides the protective, insulating layer covering many of the nerves in the body.

Use organic where possible so as to avoid the chemicals used to promote growth and control disease in crops.

Pinhead oatmeal porridge is an excellent, almost complete food source and great for the health of the bowel. (Soak overnight and make as for any porridge). Pinhead oatmeal has a deep cleansing effect on the colon wall. It is also one of the foods that is very good at helping to control cholesterol. It is very filling and satisfying and one doesn't feel hungry for hours afterwards. It is a very good way of supplying energy as the carbohydrates are broken down to sugar slowly over hours, giving the blood a steady supply of fuel. Many other cereals commonly eaten have been stripped of their nutrients during processing and may have inferior synthetic nutrients added instead. Also their carbohydrate content is in the form of refined sugar which enters the bloodstream very quickly thereby stressing the pancreas to produce a lot of insulin in a hurry. This leaves one prone to sugar imbalances, and adult onset diabetes is occurring at a much younger age nowadays as the pancreas is overworked producing more insulin than it was designed to do.(6)

If you drink alcohol, limit your intake. Alcohol in moderation can be beneficial to your health, but excess intake is definitely hazardous to health. Our public health experts have come to the general consensus that women should not consume more than two standard drinks daily, and men not consume more than four standard drinks daily.

(For more information on healthy eating see my recommendations in **"Guideline for Healthy Eating"** in Appendix 1).

Slow dietary change:

Some of you may want to completely overhaul your diet, but if you make the changes too abruptly you're likely to resent them and you'll probably build up cravings for various beloved foods that you've banished from your diet.

While some people can make large, abrupt changes in their lives, most find slow change easier to adapt to, and more likely to last. For example, if you suddenly stop cooking with salt and refrain from adding it at the table, you're likely to find your foods unpalatable. But if you gradually cut back on the amount of salt you use, you'll hardly notice the difference.

A diet high in fruits and vegetables provides the nutrients your body needs for energy and maintenance. Aim for at least five servings of fruits and vegetables daily.

A diet high in fruits and vegetables provides the nutrients your body needs for energy and maintenance. Aim for at least five servings of fruits and vegetables daily.

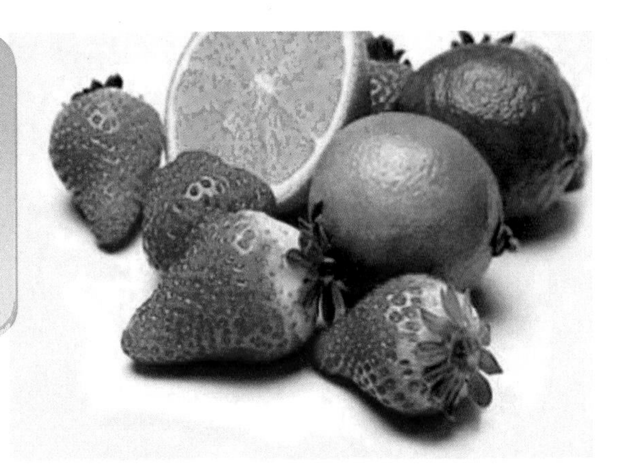

In conclusion:

Maintaining a healthy diet is really not that hard. Dietary changes can be made slowly to become part of everyday life rather than an all-out effort that burns out after a short time. Simple things like selecting a salad sandwich for lunch rather than a fried or high fat alternative; drinking water instead of fizzy drinks; opting for fruit snacks rather than biscuits or cakes and pastries can make all the difference. Also, eating lots of different nutritious foods makes a healthy diet more interesting; remember there are more fruits than just apples and oranges, and more grains than wheat!

Food has long been, and should continue to be a great source of enjoyment. You don't necessarily have to give up everything you now love to eat in order to protect your health. Just start practising discretion and moderation in your food choices. And when you adopt this new pattern of eating, the great thing you'll notice will be the surge of energy you begin to experience. Not only will you feel better, but as you nourish your body adequately, things like weight loss occur as a consequence. So eating for health can and should be very pleasurable and for more reasons than just taste.

CHAPTER 2

MODERN CIVILISATION DISEASES

> *"We don't catch diseases, we create them by breaking down the natural defences according to the way we eat, drink, think and live"*
> *- Bernard Jensen D.C., N.D.*

The central theme of this book is based on the premise that chronic low-grade inflammation is waging a silent war in your body that leads to the development of modern civilisation diseases, and that by eliminating this harmful inflammation from the body, one can ultimately regain optimal health.

Before we get deeper into the discussion on inflammation, it's important to point out that not all inflammation is bad or disease causing. There are basically two types of inflammation:

1. **Acute inflammation**
2. **Chronic inflammation**

What is Inflammation?

A standard medical dictionary defines inflammation as: "A local response to cellular injury that results in capillary dilation, immune system component infiltration, redness, heat and pain, all of which serves as a mechanism for initiating the elimination of noxious agents and damaged tissue".

In other words, in the aftermath of an injury or infection, the body's immune system initiates an inflammatory response by releasing white blood cells along with a cascade of pro-inflammatory compounds to clear out infection and damaged tissue, and then turning them off again with anti-inflammatory compounds when the threat has been neutralized. Inflammation is part of the body's defence and healing response, which acts to kill invaders, remove damaged cells and rebuild tissue. It's the body's way of combating anything that causes damage such as viruses, bacteria, allergens, toxic agents or injury.

We are all familiar with acute inflammation, the kind that protects and heals the body after an injury or infection. The redness, swelling and pain associated with acute inflammation is the result of a complex biochemical cascade of events set in motion by the body's immune system in its attempt to rid the body of either toxins, foreign invaders or to repair and heal itself following a physical injury. It's an amazing process that on the surface just looks like swelling and usually hurts, but underneath a lot of activity is taking place; it is all part of the healing process and making things better. Acute inflammation is short-lived and self-limiting.

However, when inflammation continues for too long or is excessive or uncontrolled, it will become destructive and lead to chronic inflammatory conditions. This chronic inflammation, also known as low-grade or systemic inflammation, occurs as a result of an ongoing imbalance of many of the body's regulatory molecules involved in the inflammatory response. This unrelenting inflammatory response initiated by the body's immune system is now being considered by many researchers to be the root cause of most chronic diseases some of which I have already mentioned.

Although experts in this field of research agree it usually takes years of ongoing low-grade chronic inflammation to trigger these types of disease, there are often subtle short-term health consequences including ongoing fatigue, indigestion, mood disorders, aches and pains, and weight gain to name a few.

This revolutionary medical hypothesis can now explain hereto medical conundrums such as why high blood pressure puts patients at increased risk of Alzheimer's or why rheumatoid arthritis sufferers have higher rates of heart attack. They all seem to be connected on some fundamental level, could it be they all share in the one common trait: persistent low-grade chronic inflammation?(7) Well, the scientific world is pointing the finger from all directions at this explanation.

Causes of low-grade Inflammation

The best way to treat low-grade inflammation is to first target the cause. You will never be free of this or any other health condition without first understanding the cause. This typically is different for everybody as we are all unique individuals. As a Naturopath in the field of holistic medicine, my job is to find those inflammatory triggers unique to each person, and to see how the various dietary, lifestyle, environmental or systemic factors play their role in spinning the immune system out of balance, leading to a host of chronic illnesses.

So let's take a closer look at the reasons why the body's immune system goes into overdrive causing it to get permanently stuck in the inflammation mode. Once we know the causes and remove them, we'll be in a better position to help reset the body's natural immune balance and reverse chronic inflammation and its destructive effects.

Thankfully, the list of things that cause inflammation is relatively short. They include a range of dietary, lifestyle and systemic factors. Here are some of the major ones:

1. **Dietary Factors** – mostly white sugar, processed foods, pro-inflammatory fats such as hydrogenated (trans) fats and excess omega-6 fatty acid intake.
2. **Low-grade chronic infections** – caused by viruses, bacteria, fungi and parasites.
3. **Environmental toxins** including air, water, food and soil pollutants.
4. **Internal Dysbiosis** – producing endo-toxins as a result of disordered metabolism, or imbalanced gut bacteria.
5. **Food sensitivity** – including food allergy and food intolerances
6. **Lifestyle factors** such as: -
   - Lack of exercise (or very excessive exercise, e.g. marathon running).
   - Excessive stress
   - Lack of sleep
7. **Obesity.**
8. **Injury.**
9. **Over-acidic body pH** (Low-Grade Metabolic Acidosis).

Let's examine each of the above factors in more detail starting with poor diet and see how each are linked to inflammation

Inflammatory Response

The inflammatory response is a complex process through which many parts of the body overcome the stress of wounds and return the body to homeostasis. The primary function of the inflammatory response is to bring phagocytic cells (neutrophils and monocytes) to the inflamed area to destroy bacteria and rid the tissue spaces of dead and dying cells so that tissue repair can begin. The illustrations below trace the steps of the inflammatory response.

Inflammation produces four cardinal signs: redness, swelling, heat, and pain. The first three signs result from local vasodilation, fluid leakage into the extravascular space, and blockage of lymphatic drainage. The fourth results from tissue space distention caused by swelling and pressure, and from chemical irritation of nociceptors (pain receptors).

The acute phase of the inflammatory response typically lasts 2 weeks; the subacute phase (a less intense version of the acute phase), 2 weeks.

(1) Splinter punctures epidermis
(2) Bacteria introduced
(3) Bacteria implanted in tissue
(4) Injured cells release histamine and kinins, causing capillary dilation
(5) Dilated capillaries make skin hot and red; escaping fluid from blood vessels causes swelling; edema, kinins, and other substances produce pain; neutrophils and monocytes migrate through vessel walls toward bacteria
(6) Neutrophils and monocytes destroy bacteria by phagocytosis

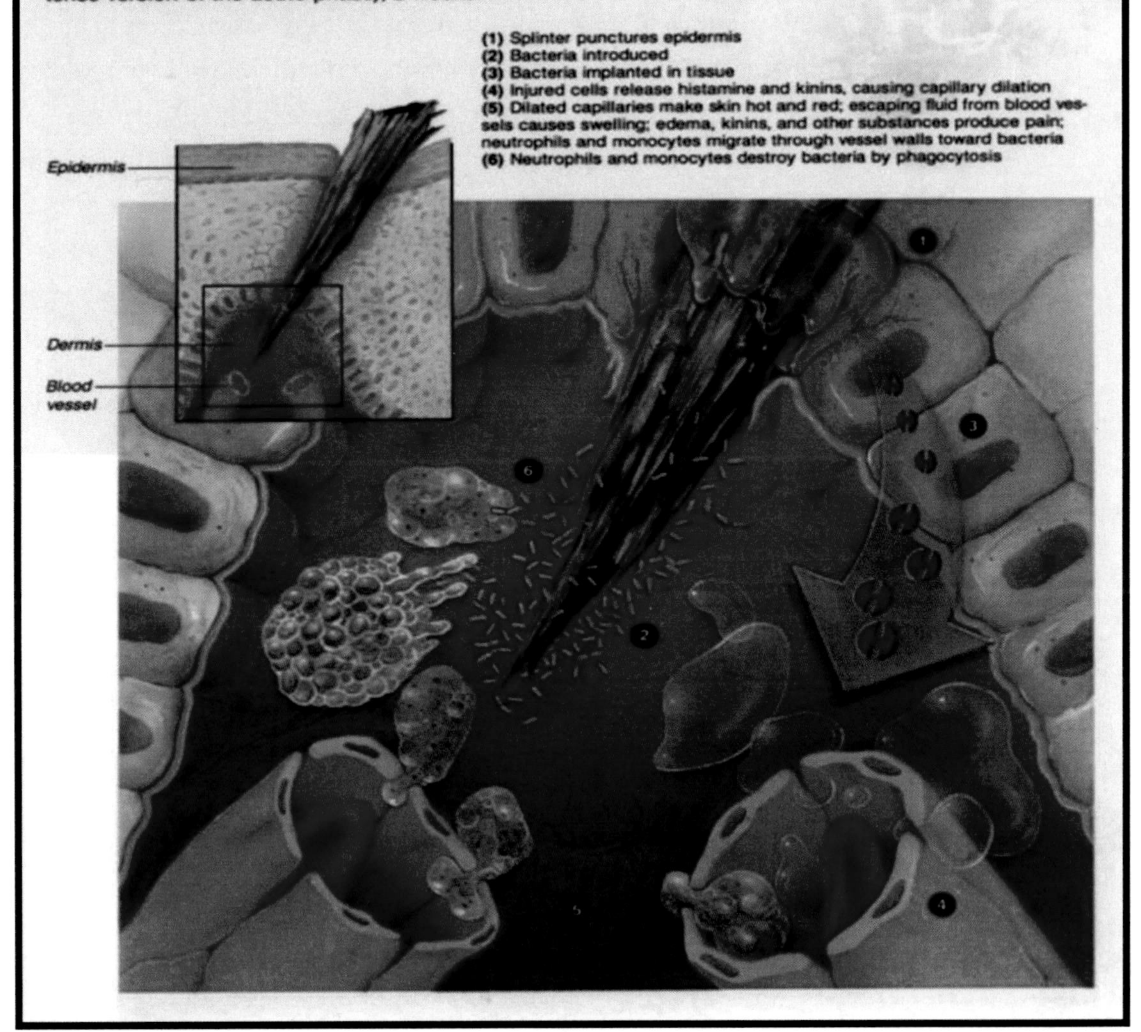

1. Dietary Factors

Of all of the contributing factors to inflammation, a poor diet stands out as a primary cause. Our typical modern diet of refined, over-processed and denatured foods contains vastly increased amount of disease-inducing pro-inflammatory nutrients compared to the typical diet of 50 to 100 years ago. As a result, people have biochemically primed their bodies for ongoing inflammation, which can then be triggered more easily by other contributing factors.

We've all heard about omega-3 & omega-6 oils and how essential they are for our health. Unfortunately with today's diet, our intake of these oils is quite imbalanced with the average person consuming a much higher ratio of 6 to 3 omega oils thereby contributing to increased inflammation inside their body.(8) It's not that omega-6 oils are bad for you, they are actually needed in small amount for essential uses, but if you eat too many omega-6s and not enough omega-3s, it creates an imbalance in the body's chemistry leading to inflammation. Excess consumption of omega-6 oils have been shown to contribute to many chronic and life-threatening conditions including cancer, heart disease, immune dysfunction, liver damage and obesity.(8) Other organs adversely affected include the reproductive organs, lungs, brain and digestive system.

Omega-6 oils are found in abundance in polyunsaturated vegetable oils such as sunflower, grape seed, safflower, canola, soybean and corn oil. They can get converted into arachidonic acid, which in turn gets converted into pro-inflammatory compounds known as Series-2 prostaglandins or PG2 Series; whose job it is to enhance the inflammatory process.

Omega-3 oils on the other hand are found in cold water fish including salmon, mackerel, trout, herring, tuna and sardines. Plant sources include flaxseeds, walnuts, almonds, cashews and acai berries. The omega-3 essential fatty acids through a series of biochemical processes, gets converted into Series-3 prostaglandins (PG3 Series) that quell the inflammatory response.

Hydrogenation:-

The process called hydrogenation is where hydrogen atoms are forced into polyunsaturated oils under high pressure and temperature in order to turn the oils into fatty solids. These fatty solids are then made into margarines, shortening, and used widely in the confectionary industry. The oils get changed at the molecular level during the hydrogenation process resulting in the creation of trans-fatty acids. These trans-fatty acids do not occur in nature and so cannot be properly metabolised and used within the body.

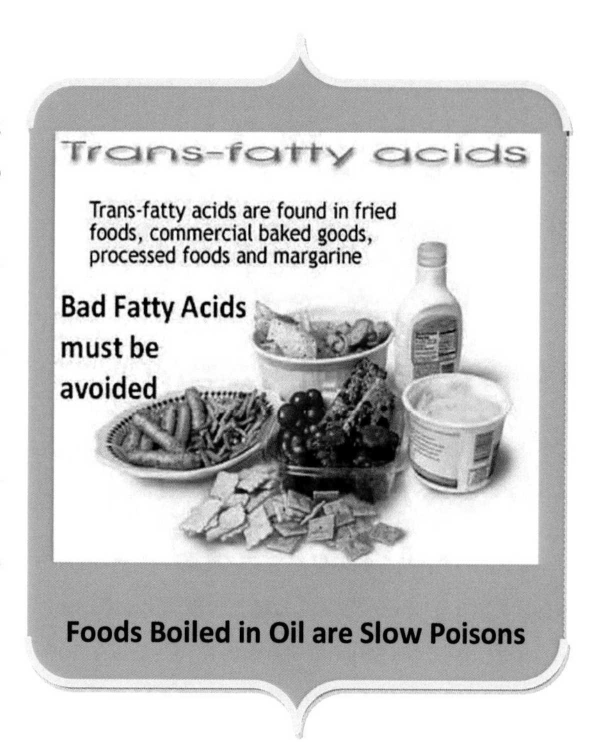

Foods Boiled in Oil are Slow Poisons

However, these man-made toxins end up being incorporated into cell membranes where they can cause havoc with cell metabolism. They block the proper utilization of essential fatty acids, thereby inducing cellular dysfunction and promote ongoing inflammation.(9) Not only has the consumption of hydrogenated (trans) fats been implicated in heart disease and cancer, but also, a host of other conditions such as sexual dysfunction, high cholesterol, diabetes, obesity, birth defects, immune disorders, deteriorating eyesight, sterility and bone problems.(10)

The newer margarines, while lower in hydrogenated fats, are still made from cheaply-produced rancid vegetable oils such as soy, corn, canola or rapeseed and contain many additives. Your best defence is to avoid all hydrogenated products like the plague.

Foods that are high in arachidonic acid include red meats (especially organ meats), also dairy products; and should only be consumed in small quantities as they are promoters of inflammation. The reason being, arachidonic acid, through a number of biochemical pathways, gets converted into the pro-inflammatory Series-2 prostaglandins.

Sugar and High Glycaemic Index Foods:

The term High Glycaemic Index refers to foods that quickly raise blood sugar levels when ingested. Sugar and highly refined foods along with some fruits, tend to have a higher glycaemic index than unprocessed and complex carbohydrate foods. Foods that quickly raise your blood sugar levels cause your pancreas to over-react and excrete unusually high amounts of insulin to quickly normalise blood sugar levels again. This results in excessive glucose concentration within tissue cells that can promote the formation of Advanced Glycosylation End Products (AGEs).

AGE's are produced when a protein is bound to a glucose molecule, resulting in damaged cross-linked proteins. (Cross-linking is how wrinkles are formed) AGE's in turn generate huge amounts of free radicals that damage cellular structures. As our bodies try to dismantle these AGEs, immune cells are activated to release lots of pro-inflammatory compounds called cytokines that promote inflammation. This glycation can result in many negative effects including thickened arteries, stiff joints, weak muscles and failing organs.

Food cooked at a high temperature as in frying, roasting and barbequed food also create AGEs, a fact worth remembering when it comes to methods of food preparation. The deleterious effects of AGEs are most evident in diabetics whom we know suffer from high levels of inflammation and free radical damage. Their hyperglycaemia state is primarily attributable to the formation of high amounts of AGEs. As a result, diabetic patients commonly suffer from many complications including retinal damage leading to blindness, kidney damage, cardiovascular disease including heart attacks and strokes and increased risk of cancers. These complications are a direct result of the systemic inflammation and free radical damage caused by the over-production of AGEs.

This clear connection associating excessive sugar intake with the promotion of inflammation within the body has been demonstrated by numerous studies over recent years. In 2013 a damning report from the Credit Suisse's Research Institute in

America revealed the dire health consequences of consuming excessive sugar. The report highlighted several health conditions including heart disease, type 2 diabetes and metabolic syndrome (a pre-diabetic condition) that numerous studies have previously linked to excessive sugar intake.(11)

Robert Lustig, an endocrinologist from California, investigated the connection between sugar consumption and poor health, found conclusive evidence that excessive sugar intake plays a key role in the etiology of many types of cancer, coronary heart disease and hypertension, as well as type 2 diabetes and obesity. He concluded that 75% of all diseases are the result of our modern diet and as such are entirely preventable.(12)

The damaging effects of sugar on brain function have been well researched in recent years. A 2012 article entitled "Food for Thought: Eat Your Way to Dementia", American researchers from Brown University presented their findings that a diet high in sugar disrupts insulin levels that may trigger the build-up of toxic amyloid proteins – the proteins directly implicated in the progression of dementia in the brain.(13)

These conclusions are backed up by another study carried out by the Mayo Clinic in 2012, which showed that seniors who consumed a diet high in sugars and refined carbohydrates had a much greater risk of developing dementia when compared to seniors whose diet contained more proteins and fats.

Again, numerous studies show a direct relationship between sugar consumption and the risk of cancer. As far back as the 1930's Otto Warburg MD, a Nobel laureate in medicine, discovered that cancer cells could only survive on a steady supply of glucose. The more primitive nature of cancer cells means these cells are not able to synthesize glucose from larger molecules. Their reliance on glucose as their source of fuel gives rise to a build-up of lactic acid from direct consumption of glucose by cancer cells. This creates an acidic pH and is a diagnostic factor for cancer.(14)

So now you know why diets high in sugar and refined foods are so harmful to everyone, not just diabetics. Your best bet is to eat more whole grains, brown rice, vegetables and legumes in their natural state so as to prevent after-meal sugar spikes, thereby reducing the formation of AGEs and resultant cytokine production.

Appendix 2 at the back of the book has a list of anti-inflammatory versus pro-inflammatory foods and the ideal ratios to eat them.

2. Infections

It has been long known that bacteria, viruses, fungal infections and parasites cause low-grade inflammation. For instance, the common bacterium Helicobacter pylorus that affects the stomach induces inflammation in the stomach mucosa that can lead to ulcers and even stomach cancer.

Anti-candida Treatment

To prevent or help cure candidiasis, crush one clove of garlic (a segment of the bulb) and take immediately, either mixed with natural yoghurt, mashed potatoes or mashed vegetables, or mixed with olive oil and poured over a salad. Wash down with a glass of water afterwards and do this three times per day during meals.

Women who suffer from repeated bouts of cystitis (urinary tract infections) caused by bacteria will have chronically inflamed bladders, which puts them at increased risk of developing squamous-cell bladder cancer. In some areas of the planet, this type of cancer is linked to chronic inflammation caused by infection with a parasite.

Candida Albicans is an unfriendly fungus (also referred to as a yeast) which commonly resides in the gastrointestinal tract. Ordinarily, our friendly gut bacteria keeps candida levels in check, but when various factors come into play such as consuming a diet high in sugars and processed foods, antibiotic use (kills friendly bacteria), taking the contraceptive pill, or having health conditions like diabetes or obesity, then candida levels can drastically rise, causing a condition called Candidiasis.

This Candidiasis (overgrowth of Candida Albicans) is believed to be a major underlying factor in a host of conditions including inflammatory bowel disease, gastritis, Crohn's disease, ulcerative colitis, and gastric and duodenal ulcers, all due to its pro-inflammatory promoting characteristics. When candida grows unchecked, it changes its form, from a spore into a mycelia form which puts down roots and spreads rapidly. These roots are able to penetrate the intestinal wall causing a leaky gut that allows partially digested food, toxic waste, etc. to enter the blood stream resulting in allergies and a continual drain on the immune system.

Because of the damage to the mucosal lining of the digestive tract wrought by candida overgrowth, this fungus can then enter the blood stream, which leads to fungal candida setting up throughout the body. The effects can be devastating, causing a myriad of symptoms including chronic fatigue, skin rashes, sinusitis, asthma, thrush, joint pains, depression and mood swings, cravings (specifically for alcohol, bread and sweets), autoimmune diseases and many more.

Here is a simple Candida yeast test you can do in the morning

As soon as you awake in the morning and before you put anything into your mouth, work up some saliva and spit it into a clear glass of water. Within a couple of minutes look in the glass to see if there are strings coming down from your saliva, or if the water has turned cloudy, or if your saliva has sank to the bottom of the glass, **YOU MAY HAVE A CANDIDA PROBLEM!** Healthy saliva will simply float on the top! (See **Appendix 3** for an Anti-candida dietary programme to follow if you have candida overgrowth).

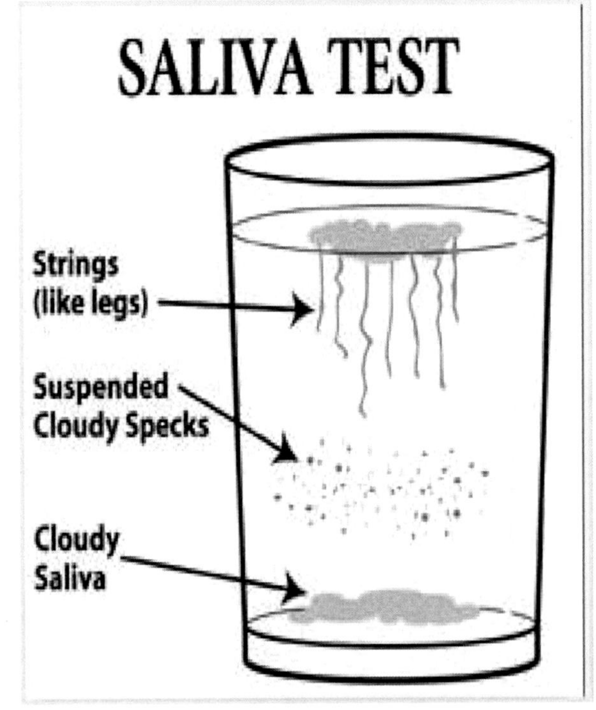

Poor dental health can be another cause of systemic inflammation. Researchers have made direct connections between periodontal (gum) disease and cardio-vascular disease.(15) Bacteria from bleeding gums can enter the bloodstream and damage the heart valves and also the endothelial lining of arteries, causing inflammation, which subsequently leads to clogging of arteries and eventual heart failure.

Parasites:

The very name may send shivers up and down your spine. There are more parasites than any other living thing on this planet by volume. This truly is the planet of the worms and we are just symbiotic creatures trying to live in harmony with them. These little pests are everywhere; in the air you breath, your food chain, the water you drink, your darling pets and also in you my friend! Yes! We all have parasites in our bodies from time to time and those of us with weaker immune systems may permanently house these little critters.

A parasite is an organism that lives inside our bodies feeding off our body cells and the food we eat. They invariably produce waste-toxins; they damage our cells and play havoc with our immune system causing inflammation and disease. Some examples of parasites that can get into your body include Tapeworms, Pinworms and Hookworms (See next page).

We pick up parasites in a number of ways: The main source is eating undercooked meats followed by household pets when we allow them lick us. You can get parasites from drinking contaminated water, from eating vegetables and salads when not properly washed; even from inhaling dust that contains the dried spores of these organisms. Other modes of entry include sharing utensils, kissing and intimate contact and even breast feeding mothers can pass them on to their babies.

Once inside the body, parasites proliferate quite rapidly! They can take up residence anywhere in your body; from your gut to your liver, lungs, skin, even our eyes and brain can be infiltrated.

The most common symptom of parasite infestation is fatigue due to the fact that these little monsters are busily feeding off both your body tissues and also your food supply depriving you of important nutrients. Indeed, the list of symptoms one suffers is often so wide and diverse that the underlying parasitic cause usually goes undiagnosed and therefore inappropriate treatment is given.

With parasitic infestation, one can suffer from the usual digestive complaints (i.e. gas, bloating, heartburn, constipation or diarrhoea), itchy anus, nose or ears, foggy thinking, headaches, mood disorders, blurry vision, joint pains, fluid retention, poor libido, inexplicable chills and fever, or autoimmune diseases, to name but a few. Unless these parasites are properly dealt with and fully eliminated from your body, you will continue to suffer ill health. I have found herbal formulas with cloves, goldenrod, goldenseal root, Black walnut hulls, Wormwood, Tansey, Olive leaf, Pumpkin seeds, anise seeds, cayenne, turmeric, garlic and thymus are very effective in killing parasites and their eggs. The use of such herbs in a parasite cleansing programme can flush out the worms and effectively de-worm the adult or child. We all need to de-worm at least once a year and not allow parasites to over proliferate.

The following pictorial gallery shows what a few of the commonly known invading parasites look like, and that may also call the human body their home...

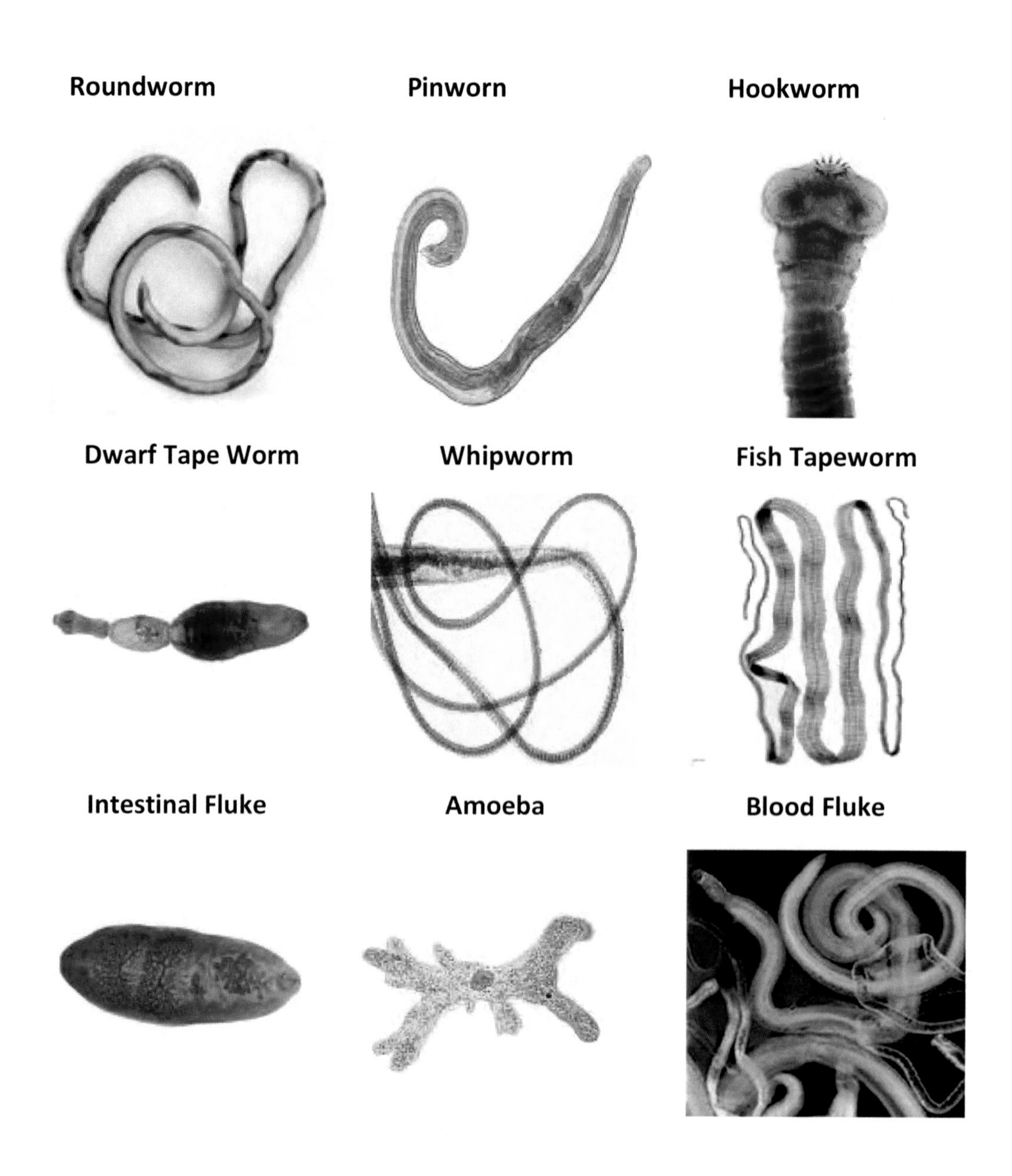

3. Environmental Toxins

We live in a poisoned world. Thousands upon thousands of dangerous chemicals enter the environment everyday whereupon they can freely enter our bodies and interfere with our hormonal system, nervous system and immune system triggering ongoing inflammation and affecting metabolic functions and ultimately promoting the development of chronic disease within our bodies

Most foreign substances enter the body via the skin, lungs or digestive tract. Generally referred to as "Exotoxins", these substances originate outside of the body as opposed to "Endotoxins", which are substances produced from within the body as a consequence of imbalanced metabolism and microbial activity.

Air, water, food and soil pollutants are the source of most exotoxins. The exhaust fumes from cars, factories and power plants contaminate the air we breathe. Chlorine, fluoride, arsenic, lead and a host of industrial wastes pollute our water. Pesticides, herbicides and countless other noxious chemicals are used in our food supply that it's estimated the average person consumes nearly a gallon of these chemicals each year.(16) In fact, nearly everything we eat has either been preserved, dipped, dyed or sprayed. And as if that's not enough, we rub chemical cosmetics on our skin, and when not feeling well, rely on chemical drugs to make us better!

The presence of many of these exotoxins in the body has been positively linked with specific diseases and syndromes. For instance, we know that in areas where air pollution is heaviest as in large town and cities, the incidence of respiratory illnesses such as asthma and bronchitis increases. We know smokers have a much greater risk of getting cancer, heart disease and strokes than non-smokers. Their constant exposure to tobacco toxins elicits an ongoing immune response that generates storms of free radicals and other pro-inflammatory cytokines that damage body cells and arterial walls leading to the inevitable.

The greatest sources of air pollution originate from the waste combustion pollutants of burning fossil fuels, factory and power generation wastes, traffic fumes and smoking. Serious health problems can and do result from these pollutants.

Recent studies have shown that people exposed to pesticides have a much higher incidence of both Parkinson's and Alzheimer's disease. These studies revealed that pesticides activate specialised immune cells in the brain called microglia resulting in chronic localized inflammation. The trouble is that these microglia cells are highly concentrated in the parts of the brain responsible for Parkinson's and Alzheimer's disease.(17)

"Pesticide"! What does that mean? Well "cide" means "to kill" and "pest" is self-explanatory, so pesticide means to kill pests. Pesticides are used so as to grow crops at a more profitable rate. The downside is that residues of these pesticides are going into our bodies and in the same way that it kills the DNA and disrupts the immune system of the pest; it also does similar harm to our bodies!

National Geographic in the October 2005 issue reported that there are over 82,000 unregulated man-made chemicals in production today and only a quarter of them have ever been tested for toxicity.(18) Over 3,000 chemicals can be found in the average home. It's been confirmed that indoor air pollution is more damaging to the body, circulating from carpets, furniture, heating systems, wall paint, cleaning agents and moulds. There are over 3,500 chemicals used in the food supply. Many are unregulated chemicals such as preservatives, colouring agents, and flavouring agents. Some experts suggest that our exposure to these chemicals causes 80% of all cancers. These toxins have also been linked to chronic degenerative diseases including heart disease, diabetes and autoimmune diseases. They can also cause us to gain weight, suffer reproductive problems, experience depression, aggression and memory loss.

While it would be impossible to eliminate all chemical exotoxins, there are things you can do to reduce exposure and lessen their impact. You can avoid pesticides, herbicides, antibiotics and synthetic hormones by eating an organic diet. You can drink only filtered or distilled water; I personally use a reverse osmosis filter that eliminates up to 99% of chemicals from my drinking water. You can use natural plant-based cosmetics instead of synthetic chemical-based ones. You can clean your home with natural cleaners such as vinegar and baking soda, and reduce the amount of dust and mould spores in your house by vacuuming and using an ozone generator

OZONE GENERATOR

Ozone generators are small electrical devices that produce ozone gas, which can be used for cleaning the air we breathe and also, for purifying and oxygenating the water we drink.

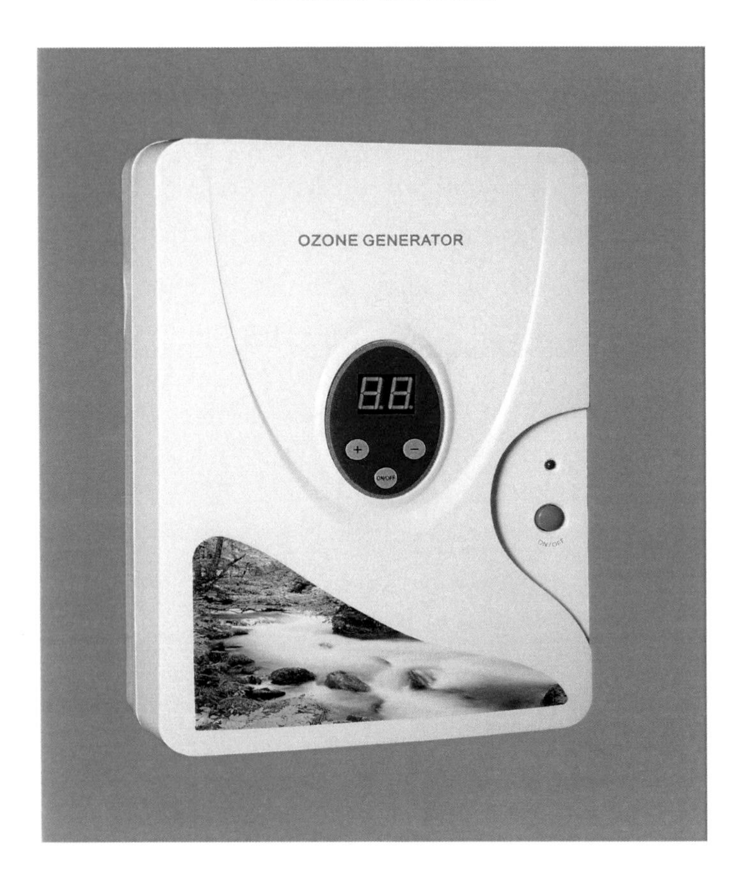

What is Ozone?

Ozone is a molecule composed of three atoms of oxygen. Two atoms of oxygen form the basic oxygen molecule--the oxygen we breathe that is essential to life.

The third oxygen atom can detach from the ozone molecule, and this singlet oxygen atom is HIGHLY REACTIVE with just about any substance it comes into contact with. In chemical terms ozone is an oxidizer. In simpler terms it destroys bacteria, viruses, parasites, moulds, fungus, and also breaks down harmful chemicals and toxins.

Ozonated Water

Ozonated water is highly beneficial to both healthy and sickly people. It's easy to make and should be consumed regularly. Besides providing more oxygen to the body cells, ozonated water will oxidize toxins and kill pathogens in the body, allowing for their complete elimination through excretion.

To make ozonated water using the generator pictured (these can be purchased at my clinic), simply place the output tubing with the attached air stone bubbler into a large glass or pitcher filled with water (preferably filtered) and run the machine for 10 minutes. The ozone will still oxidize out any undesirable contaminants if you use tap water.

Airborne Pathogens

Ozone can also eliminate odours and disease causing pathogens that travel through the air and have the potential to affect everyone. Using the ozone generator every day keeps the air fresh and clean in your home. I personally use the Ozone Generator every day to help improve my health and general well-being. As well as drinking ozonated water I also use it to purify and refresh the air in my office and home by having it on for 30 minutes each day.

4. Internal Dysbiosis

The term dysbiosis was coined in the early 20th Century by Dr. Eli Metchnikoss. By combining the root word "dys" (meaning abnormal, bad, or ill) with the word "symbiosis" (meaning the living together in harmony between two different organisms), we get the word Dysbiosis, which means "not living together in harmony". So, internal dysbiosis essentially relates to the imbalance of good versus bad bacteria within the body.

Dysbiosis occurs most notably in the gastrointestinal tract where there is an abundance of micro-flora, but it can also occur elsewhere on the body where there are colonies of bacteria living, such as the skin, nose, sinuses, ears, lungs, nails and vagina.

Our bodies are very much akin to a finely tuned ecosystem where it is estimated that the numbers of bacteria living within our body outnumber human cells by a ratio of10:1.(19) In other words, the human body is home to more than 500 trillion bacteria with a combined weight of approximately 3kg of these tiny single-celled organisms.

We will only experience optimal health and vitality when we are co-existing in a friendly symbiotic relationship with this micro-flora that inhabits our bodies. These microbial colonies excrete many different types of waste by-products, some beneficial and some potentially toxic to their host. However, health problems can occur when there is a shift in the balance of good and bad bacteria. When there is an overpopulation of unfriendly bacteria in the host, these bacteria shed endotoxins, which slowly enter the bloodstream setting the stage for immune activation and consequent low-grade systemic inflammation to occur. (Endotoxins refer to toxins produced inside the body either through microbial activity or imbalanced metabolism).

Using different waste removal systems, our bodies can safely neutralize these by-products. However, when your system is overwhelmed by the increased number of pathogenic or bad bacteria producing increased amount of these toxic by-products, our body's elimination systems become overloaded and malfunctions. These toxins then seep into the body tissues causing cellular disruption and immune activation thereby setting the stage for chronic inflammation and degenerative diseases to occur.

From my many years of clinical experience working in the Naturopathic field of medicine, I've discovered that the root cause of so many health problems of today are the result of microbial dysbiosis, primarily originating in the gastrointestinal tract. Unfortunately, most people have never heard of the concept of disharmony in gut micro-flora and so carry on superficially treating their symptoms instead of addressing the larger issue of gut dysbiosis.

The modern diet filled with exorbitant amounts of processed and sugar-laden foods are the fuel for the unfriendly bacteria. These bacteria feed on the sugars and produce toxic by-products that ferment in the intestines, creating gas and a bloated feeling. These by-products (endotoxins) are irritants to the digestive tract, which cause an inflamed gut, facilitate the overgrowth of yeasts (candida) and contribute to a condition known as "Leaky Gut Syndrome". Gastrointestinal disorders such as irritable bowel syndrome and inflammatory bowel disease, as well as more systemic conditions such as fibromyalgia, chronic fatigue and rheumatoid arthritis can be directly attributed to gut dysbiosis.

Consistently eating high-fat and low fibre foods such as a diet based mainly on animal products, creates a slower bowel transit time. This results in increased bile acid secretion in response to the high animal fat intake. These bile acids can then get converted into more toxic secondary bile acids by pathogenic bacteria, along with an increased production of other dangerous metabolites such as ammonia, nitrites, aromatic hydrocarbons and nitrosamines, which can further irritate the digestive

Leaky Gut

Leaky Gut is a condition where there is an increase in the permeability of the lining of the intestinal tract, which results in substances such as toxins microbes and undigested food leaking from the gut into the bloodstream, resulting in ongoing inflammation.

tract to cause symptoms such as constipation, diarrhoea, headaches, aches and pains and a general overall sense of ill-health.

Low stomach acid (hydrochloric acid), which leads to improper digestion, can also promote dysbiosis. What happens is the pH of the small intestine is raised via the fermentation taking place in the stomach, thereby permitting the overgrowth of microbes within the small intestines. In addition to this, the incompletely digested food leaving the stomach is then available to nourish the unfriendly bacteria in both the small and large intestines.

Taking antacids to alleviate symptoms of heartburn only compounds the problem and contributes further to gut dysbiosis. I've found from years of clinical practice that the cause of heartburn in my clients is seldom the result of excess production of hydrochloric acid and more likely to be due to low stomach acid, which results in fermentation in the stomach and small intestine, and the resultant gaseous mixture being the underlying reason for heartburn.

In addition to low stomach acid and a poor diet, medications like antibiotics, non-steroidal anti-inflammatory drugs (NSAID's), the contraceptive pill, antacids and parasites, as well as the stressors of modern day living are all contributing factors to imbalanced bowel flora.

Ways to reduce endotoxin production particularly in the gut may be as general as encouraging a more plant-based diet with better meal patterning, smaller meals and better chewing of foods. In addition, intestinal dysbiosis can be treated with a variety of herbal medicines to rid your body of unfriendly organisms. Treatment of dysbiosis caused by bacteria and yeast overgrowth will also usually include supplementation with friendly probiotic organisms such as Lactobacillus and Bifidobacterium.

5. Food Sensitivity (Food Allergy and Food Intolerance)

When most people think of food allergies they visualise symptoms such as itchy hives and angry looking skin rashes or they imagine someone eating peanuts or shellfish and ending up in the emergency room with a swollen tongue and barely able to breathe. As a description of food allergies, this is accurate. It is a particular type of food allergy known as Type-1 IgE-mediated reaction. It can be very serious for the susceptible individual but thankfully this extreme version is not very common. Most individuals instead, tend to suffer from a delayed allergy where their symptoms are much less dramatic and deadly, but nonetheless still troublesome and ultimately can cause them serious harm.

Exposure to food allergens can trigger chronic inflammatory reactions in susceptible individuals. Even slight food intolerances can brew ongoing inflammation that leads to greater health problems and chronic disease further down the road.

Common allergies like for instance, to the proteins "casein" found in milk and "gluten" found in wheat, oats, barley and rye, are quick to spark an inflammatory cascade in susceptible individuals. Anyone suffering from coeliac disease, a digestive disorder that interferes with the absorption of nutrients from food, is painfully aware of the damaging effects of gluten containing foods.

These types of food allergy differ from food intolerances in that, symptoms are usually immediate, occurring within minutes of ingesting the offending food. Even exposure to minute quantities of the guilty allergen can set off an immediate attack. So if you are sensitive to pollen, a few grains of the dust can cause streaming, itchy eyes, a runny nose or asthma. If you are allergic to a particular food, for example, peanuts, a touch of it on your lips will make them swell, if you are unlucky enough to swallow a piece, your throat may swell and potentially choke you. Admittedly, with this particular type of immune-mediated allergy i.e. IgE, the symptoms are not always quite as dramatic and violent as this, but you are certainly left in no doubt as to the cause of the problem.

The reason for these sudden reactions are due to a group of specialized immune cells called 'Mast cells', which have become sensitized to the offending allergen. And how can this come about, you may wonder? Well, it happens in two stages: The first stage is when a susceptible individual is first exposed to the allergen. The person experiences no symptoms at all. But during this stage, their immune system has been stimulated into producing high amounts of a particular type of antibody call "Immunoglobulin E" or IgE for short, in response to the presence of the allergen.

These IgE antibodies then attach en-mass to receptors on mast cells that are typically located in the region of the body where the exposure first occurred. Mast cells being a type of immune cell contain large quantities of pro-inflammatory compounds including histamine and bradykinins along with a number of other irritating chemicals including one called slow-reacting substance of anaphylaxis. The functions of these chemicals are to increase the flow of fluids in and out of blood vessels. They increase the amounts and types of fluid produced by the mucus producing glands and they also cause involuntary muscles located throughout the body's internal organs to contract.

Now, in the normal course of events, these chemicals are being slowly released all the time to regulate our natural bodily functions. But in a sensitized individual whose mast cells have been covered by IgE antibodies, the arrival of a subsequent dose of the allergen puts those mast cells into a frenzied activity. They literally explode, releasing their contents of histamine and bradykinins along with the other pro-inflammatory chemicals contained therein. The result of this onslaught depends upon where the sensitized mast cells are located. If located in the nose, they will cause a discharge of watery mucous; around the eyes they will cause red itchy inflamed eyes with watery discharge, the typical symptoms of hay fever; in the lungs not only do the lining of the bronchial tubes become swollen and secrete mucus, but the smooth muscles in the bronchial walls constrict, narrowing the tubes and making breathing difficult as in an asthma attack.

If the mast cells are in the gut, the consequences can include painful intestinal spasms and diarrhoea. Also, local reaction at the intestinal lining with mast cells increases the permeability of the gut mucosa thereby allowing the allergen to enter the bloodstream. Here, it will interact with another type of immune cell called a basophil as well as with mast cells located in the body's tissues, again causing further release of inflammatory cytokines that produce hives and nettle rash all over the body.

If large enough quantities of the chemical, slow-reacting substance of anaphylaxis are released, then the result can be catastrophic anaphylaxis, a potentially fatal condition, which is characterised by a profound and prolonged drop in blood pressure accompanied by difficulty in breathing. This reaction is fortunately not common but sensitized individuals who do suffer from it will need emergency treatment in the form of oxygen and an adrenaline shot to revive them. The foods that most commonly cause this kind of acute reaction are fish, shellfish, eggs and peanuts.

While you may not suffer from a full-blown food allergy, it is likely that you may suffer from a food intolerance that has gone undiagnosed. Unlike food allergies that cause immediate symptoms, food intolerances, which are a form of masked allergy, have delayed reactions that are often hard to pinpoint and may lead to vague symptoms such as bloating, indigestion, irritable bowel, fatigue, clouded thinking, headaches, mood problems or muscle and joint pain. Also, if you experience any cravings or addictions to food or drink, it's more likely that you're suffering from a masked allergy to these substances.

The difficulty in identifying food intolerances lies in the fact that these reactions can occur days or even weeks after exposure to the offending substance. Recently a woman came to see me at my clinic suffering from as she put it: "foggy thinking and low energy". After taking a case history and doing my investigations, I discovered she was intolerant to eggs. She consumed eggs nearly every day in one form or another. So upon my suggestion, she removed them from her diet and within a couple of weeks both her energy and mental faculties improved greatly.

Unlike Type 1 IgE mediated food allergy, a **food intolerance** involves two other types of antibodies called immunoglobulins G and M (IgG, IgM). IgG is the antibody present in the largest amounts in the body and is the major immunoglobulin in blood, plus it can also enter tissue spaces. IgM is actually a cluster of five antibodies and due to its large size remains only in the bloodstream where in combination with a group of specialised proteins called the complement system, it acts to destroy invading bacteria.

IgG and IgM antibodies become activated as a result of a food allergen attaching itself to both body cells and also to blood cells. With this foreign passenger riding on their back, the cells attract these two antibodies, which sets off a cascade of events to destroy both the allergen and also the body and blood cells in the process. An important characteristic of both IgG and IgM antibodies is their ability to activate the complement system. This system comprises twenty or so proteins that normally circulate in the blood in an inactive form. Once activated by the allergen-antibody complex, this complement system will release pro-inflammatory cytotoxic substances that destroy not only the offending allergen but also body tissues in the process.

Now, if the immune system is not optimally functioning, but only going off at 'half-cock' so to speak, then the allergen and IgG or IgM antibodies are left locked in what's called an "Immune Complex". Once formed, these immune complexes induce a more severe inflammatory response by attracting other immune cells called macrophages and neutrophils, along with the activation of the complement system. Activation of these cells by the immune complexes release more potent inflammatory mediators inducing even more tissue damage and injury.

These nasty immune complexes can hang around in the body for years where they tend to lodge in the synovial tissue of joint cavities causing terrible joint pains as in rheumatoid arthritis. In the kidneys they can cause nephritis which is a type of inflammation that leads to recurrent kidney infections. If they get lodged in muscle tissues, the result is extreme muscle pain and debilitating fatigue as in fibromyalgia, and in the skin they will cause a raised skin rash.

Now, after reading and trying to digest all that information on food allergy and food intolerance, in order to do this section full justice, I feel it my duty to inform you about one other type of food allergy/intolerance mechanism that doesn't require the participation of antibodies. Instead, this particular hypersensitivity is due primarily to the interaction of the allergen with an immune cell called a T-cell. These T-cells are also known as memory cells and can remain in the body for years, so that individuals who have become sensitized to a particular substance tend to remain so. These T-cells can be activated every time the offending allergen is introduced into the person's diet. Once stimulated, the T-cells secrete lymphokines along with a variety of other inflammatory mediators that in turn recruit and activate a host of other immune cells, triggering an immune response with resultant inflammation.

Prevention and Treatment of Food Sensitivity

Susceptibility to an allergen depends on a number of different factors as well as heredity and the health of the body's immune system. Chief among the causes are poor diet and lifestyle habits along with medications and environmental factors. Also, leading a stressful lifestyle, insufficient sleep and underlying infections can predispose the body to developing allergies. A healthy body can resist allergens, but a deficiency in any one or more micro-nutrients can increase cell permeability allowing easy entrance by foreign substances and setting the stage for allergic reactions to occur. Also, a leaky gut allows partially digested foods get exposed to your immune system, which then creates an abnormal response to something that should otherwise be normal- i.e. food.

Another common cause of the increased incidence of allergies and intolerances, is today's processed foods have been loaded with countless additives and preservatives, flavour enhancers, colorants and many other artificial ingredients. As a general rule, those of you and indeed all of us who suffer from food sensitivities should avoid all foods that might possibly contain chemical additives or residues from pesticides and sprays and eat only organically produced foods free from chemical adulteration.

Causes of Food Allergies

Cause1: Overeating the same foods (avoid the same food for 4-5 days)

Cause 2: Intestinal permeability (Leaky Gut)

Cause3: Not enough hydrochloric acid.

Cause 4: Not enough pancreatic enzymes.

Cause 5: Intestinal dysbiosis (Bowel flora imbalance).

Food Allergy Test

There are a number of different methods in determining what foods can be causing an allergy or intolerance in a sensitized individual. Some of the tests involve taking a blood sample and testing for IgE and IgG antibodies. This is useful and can pinpoint trouble areas but it is not 100% accurate. Another method known as applied Kinesiology which uses muscle strength and weakness to test for food sensitivity, if used expertly can be of value.

The system I use for testing food sensitivities, tests the client against a data base of over 11,000 different substances including food additives and many other chemicals via a form of electro-dermal testing, which looks for abnormal electrical patterns in the body to determine what foods or chemicals are creating such electrical aberrations.

All of the above methods are useful but it still remains that the gold standard for assessment of food sensitivity remains a systematic investigation of food itself. This is best accomplished by employing the services of a competent nutritionist or naturopath who has taken the time to develop knowledge in this area.

As a first step you need to establish a hypoallergenic diet from which all suspected food allergens have been removed. Categories of commonly reactive foods are well-known and must all be removed from the diet for a period of at

The Ten Major Food Allergens

1. Dairy products – milk and cheese in particular

2. Wheat – the sensitivity may be either to gluten or to other components of the grain.

3. Eggs

4. Nuts – most notably peanuts, but also almonds, cashews and walnuts.

5. Vegetable of the Solanacae family which include potatoes, tomatoes, eggplant, peppers and chillies.

6. Shellfish such as prawns, crabs, lobster and oysters.

7. Fish, especially cod and salmon.

8. Salicylate containing foods especially strawberries and all berries that are high in salicylates.

9. Artificial food additives such as sulphites as well as other preservatives, colourings and flavourings (e.g. MSG)

10. Soyabean products.

least three to four weeks. Less well known are the seemingly infinite numbers of hiding places for these same potential allergens in the food supply. Food labels cannot be relied upon to fully inform you of a product's composition. Again, the help of a competent naturopath or dietician who has developed specific skills in this area is often essential.

Most people get into the habit of regularly consuming the same foods day after day, many of which are common causes of food sensitivities. Remember what I said earlier about food cravings and addictions being probable allergens. This repeated exposure greatly increases your chances of developing a sensitivity to a particular food or beverage.

As a general rule to lowering your risk of developing food sensitivities you should make it a habit to eat a wide variety of foods and also rotate these foods so as not to eat the same foods from day to day.

In addition to eliminating the well-known categories of reactive foods like wheat, dairy, eggs, etc, while on

- **High Salicylate Foods**
- **Fruits**: - apricots, cherries, blueberries, strawberries, raspberries, blackcurrants, cranberry, grapes, plums, sultanas, raisins, oranges, pineapple, rock melon, dates.
- **Vegetables:** - cucumber, broccoli, courgette, capsicum, eggplant, radish, tomato, peppers, sweet potato, spinach, watercress.
- **Nuts:**- almond, Brazil, macadamia, pine, pistachio, peanuts.
- **Oils:**- coconut oil, olive oil, sesame oil, walnut oil.
- **Seasonings:**- black pepper, cayenne, chilli powder, ginger, mustard, mints, nutmeg, oregano, rosemary, peppermint, sage, turmeric, vinegar, yeast extract.

- **High Amine Foods**
- **Vegetables**: - spinach, tomato, eggplant, mushrooms, sauerkraut.
- **Dairy**:- aged cheeses like cheddar and Swiss, soft chesses like Brie, Danish blue, Gruyere, Parmesan and Mozzarella.
- **Fish and Meats**:- all preserved animal products including smoked, salted or pickled meat and fish; canned tuna and sardines, anchovies, all offal products, sausages.
- **Beverages**:- beer, red wines, port, sherry, cola products, cocoa.
- **Sweets**:- white and dark chocolate cocoa products.

the hypoallergenic diet, it may be necessary to exclude two other categories of foods that have been known to cause adverse reactions. These two categories are salicylate containing foods and foods high in amines. Salicylates are especially plentiful in certain fruits and seasonings while amines are present in a wide range of foods.

You will find a suitable hypoallergenic diet in Appendix 4 to follow during the elimination phase when you remove all the common allergens. You will need to stay on this diet for a period of at least three weeks and preferable four weeks before you start slowly reintroducing back into your diet the foods you've been avoiding.

The reason being, you need to allow the time necessary for all food allergens to be fully purged from your body and also to allow sufficient time for the disappearance of the many symptoms that go hand in hand with food sensitivities. For example, in relation to food cravings and addictions, when you stop taking your favourite foods and drinks you will most likely experience withdrawal symptoms much akin to an alcoholic who experiences the DT's, or a smoker suffering neurological distress when trying to kick the habit. The reason why you keep craving bread, pizza and pasta is because your body doesn't break gluten down properly and the resultant particles are chemically similar to opiates.(20) They cause a reaction in your brain that calms you down until they are gone – then the anxiety sets in as in withdrawal symptoms making your body crave more.

Generally most people won't experience such extremes when embarking on an elimination diet; rather they may suffer fatigue, headaches and out-of-sorts for a few days. Most symptoms should be well and truly gone by the end of the second week provided that the hypoallergenic diet one is on does not contain any other food sensitivities.

Although some individuals may elect to eliminate only one or two suspected foods from their diet for a period to see how they feel, this approach can yield some helpful results; however, such a method lacks the control necessary to clearly identify all allergenic foods. Neither, does it allow for a proper challenge phase to test for an allergenic response, and so for this reason I prefer a total elimination diet as the gold standard and best method of testing for all food sensitivities.

In designing the low-reactive elimination diet, I have laid it out in such a way that if correctly followed you would not consume the same foods on a daily basis. Instead a different group of foods are eaten each of the days and then the cycle is repeated. So if you eat beans one day, don't eat beans again for the next few days. If you eat fish on a particular day, wait a few days before consuming the same fish again.

It is essential that no food be ingested more often than every three to four days so as not to develop sensitivity to any of the foods in the elimination diet. As I have previously stated, if you consume the same foods daily, your body builds up an intolerance to them. Rather than nourishing the body, such foods can instead cause harmful reactions. It can take up to four days for a food to be fully eliminated from the body and possibly even longer if one tends to suffer from constipation.

Once you have been on the elimination phase of the diet for a sufficient time (when all symptoms disappear), you can then start the challenge phase where you re-introduce back into your diet the eliminated foods one at a time to observe for any adverse reactions.

Food sensitivity symptoms often develop slowly over time so when testing, keep in mind that you may not notice any adverse reactions for up the three days after consumption of the particular food being tested. If after three days of increasing intake, you still notice no symptoms, then you can assume that you are not sensitive to that particular food. You can then continue to eat that food in moderation as part of the rotation process, and go on to test for the next eliminated food on your list. If any symptoms do occur then the offending food must be eliminated from the diet and you carry on with the rotation diet without introducing any new foods until all symptoms have again subsided. This usually takes about three days, whereupon you can then test for the next food on your list.

For the best way of testing, it is recommended that all foods within a particular food group should be tested for before moving on to test foods in a different group. So if you test for milk, then the next food to test could be natural yoghurt, then after that test for cheese and so on until all dairy products have been tested. Only then should you start testing another food group, for example grains. So you would then start testing for wheat by consuming three Weetabix mixed in milk only if you are not intolerant to milk, otherwise take the Weetabix in water or dry, or with rice milk. Then move on to other grains like oats, barley and rye.

Again as I have stated, if you show an adverse reaction during the testing process, cease taking that tested food and stay on the rotation diet (including the previously tested foods that were deemed OK) until all symptoms have cleared before starting the next challenge test. Typically this takes at least three days.

Symptoms to look out for during the testing phase can be so varied and may affect any part of the body, so it's important to be vigilant in your observations during this phase. For instance, you many get bloated, have excess wind, suffer indigestion or get either constipation or diarrhoea. Other symptoms to watch out for include headaches, sinus congestion, spacey feeling, generalised fatigue, itchy skin, depressed feelings, or aches and pains. Some individuals may even get a rapid pulse or heart palpitations after eating an allergenic food or beverage. This list is nowhere exhaustive so these and many other symptoms that can occur during the testing phase should alert you to a probable allergenic food or substance, which then needs to be promptly removed from your diet.

Clients often ask me if they need to stay off allergenic foods forever, once discovered. The answer is sometimes. It all depends on whether their particular food sensitivity is Type 1 IgE mediated in which case it's a long-lasting allergy, so any provocation in the future usually elicits an allergenic response. For instance, once you are allergic to peanuts or bee stings, which are an IgE mediated reaction, you will always be sensitized that way, and so it is best to avoid such substances permanently.

Food sensitivities that are IgG, IGM and T-cell mediated reactions, when removed from the diet for a period of six to nine months, can usually be reintroduced in small amounts without a reoccurrence of symptoms provided such foods are rotated on a regular basis. For example, if you have previously been sensitive to pork, then when reintroduced back into your diet, eat it only once a week. Foods such as eggs or cheese may now be well-tolerated once or twice a week rather than every day.

Correcting any other underlying health conditions can also help reverse many food sensitivities. Inadequate stomach acid and digestive enzymes lead to changes in gut bacteria that in turn bring about bowel toxicity and Candida overgrowth that damages the gut's lining, causing a leaky gut. And so food particles "leak" across this damaged barrier and your immune system (60% of which is located under that lining), starts to attack these partially digested foods.

Fixing these underlying pathologies by supplementing each meal with digestive enzymes along with eating a healthy diet and taking nutrient supplements, where required, will help rebalance your digestive tract and eliminate most food sensitivities.

Steps for At Home Allergy Testing

As it turns out, it is rather easy to test for a food allergy yourself in the comfort of your own home. The simple steps required include the following:

- Avoid the suspect food for at least 4 days.
- Eat a moderate amount of the suspect food on an empty stomach which means no other food should have been consumed in the previous 2 hours (drinking water is ok).
- Measure your pulse rate (beats per minute) before, and a few minutes after eating the food in question.
- Calculate the difference in your pulse rate. If the pulse rose significantly (more than just a few beats per minute) after the suspect food was eaten, then an allergy is likely even if no other symptoms are noted.

RULES FOR THE STOMACH – important for allergies

The stomach is an important part of our anatomy. Food entering our mouths must be properly prepared for digestion. After being chewed and masticated by the mouth, the food is now sent to the stomach for further processing. The stomach mixes the food in an acid bath for further break-up of the nutrients. When the acid shifts alkaline to about 5.5 pH, the pylorus valve at the base of the stomach opens and the food is passed along to the primary digestive organ, the small intestine. Nature has provided us with an autonomic nervous system that regulates this process. This nervous system is designed to prefer muscle action over digestion. So if a threat or stress comes to us after a meal, such as a lion attack, our body will shift its energy from digestion to the muscles and we can survive by running away.

In our present society we have few lions, but our nerves can still stop digestion just as easily. When we allow the stomach to empty its contents prematurely the small intestine is over burdened. The food is not properly prepared for digestion. Then we get an increase in large undigested proteins and large undigested fats that can be absorbed into the blood and lymphatic system. They will enter the free fatty acid and amino acid pool and either clog up the lymphatic system or be used to make body cells, which will now be made of poor quality parts.

It is not much of a problem if we circumvent the stomach just now and then, but for some of the patients, this becomes a way of life. They constantly use antacids, too much liquid with meals, coffee, milk, or a variety of ways to empty the stomach too early. When the stomach empties there is a release of CCK, a hormone which has a slight euphoric effect. This and the release of the stuffy stomach feeling, intensify the addictive quality of the effect. But the long term effects on nutrition are very detrimental.

There are rules of the stomach that can maximize nutrition. The majority of my patients are partially sick because they violate the rules of the stomach. This is the key to weight loss and the healing of a host of other diseases. We are now seeing more and more evidence of what good nutrition can do. But it is not just what we eat that is important, but what we absorb. Even the best meal or nutrition can result in inappropriate nutrition if we violate the rules of the stomach. Food combining is just part of the answer. As such, different foods have different times for stomach digestion.

When the stomach is weak the signs will be craving fluids with a meal, bloating after a meal, itching skin especially the rectum, belching, and gas. The patient will have a difficult time digesting raw vegetables. They will complain that raw vegetables cannot be digested. This is not a fluke of their digestion or an inherited weakness. This is a sign of a weak stomach. They must work slowly, day by day building up their stomach by taking some vegetables as juice. Maybe even very dilute juice and slowly increasing the amount till their stomach develops the strength to process food properly. The nutrient content of fruits and vegetables is immense, and being able to break up the nutrients and stimulate absorption is needed for complete health and recovery.

The addictive quality of this problem is seen as our society more and more allows for breaking the rules of the stomach. The greater your health problems are or especially if your disease is serious the more you will need to observe the rules of the stomach. This is a must for proper healing.

RULES OF THE STOMACH

1. Fluids alone (no more than 120ml or 4oz. of fluid with a meal, or for two hours after a meal)

2. No coffee at meals (wait for 1.5 to 2 hours after or 1 hour before eating)

3. No milk with meals (wait for 1.5 to 2 hours after or 1 hour before eating)

4. Fruits alone (wait for 1.5 to 2 hours after or 1 hour before eating)

5. Melons alone (wait for 1.5 to 2 hours after or 1 hour before eating)

6. Small meal is better. Quality of nutrition not quantity

7. Slow meals. Savour, enjoy, rejoice, and celebrate the meal

8. Eat for nutrition not for stimulation. Eat when hungry, not when bored

9. Rest comfortably after eating for at least 35 to 45 min to maximize stomach function

10. Make and eat food with love and kindness, no violent or negative emotions

11. No antacids

12. Do not sleep for 3 hours after eating.

6. Lifestyle Factors that Cause Inflammation

a. Lack of Exercise (or very excessive exercise, e.g. marathon running)

The jury's in; all the experts agree that when it comes to living a sedentary life in conjunction with an overly processed diet, that these two factors alone are the major contributing reasons to developing chronic inflammation.

Multiple studies show that indulging in regular moderate exercise reduces the risk of cardiovascular disease, strokes, cognitive decline, osteoporosis and most other conditions. Exercise is especially protective against serious conditions such as Alzheimer's and Parkinson's disease as well as cancers including breast, colon and prostate. Exercise reduces pro-inflammatory compounds such as C-reactive proteins and various cytokines.(21)

It has been postulated that skeletal muscle acts like an endocrine organ by influencing the metabolism and improving immunity. Studies show that when skeletal muscles perform work, as in contracting and relaxing, they produce and release anti-inflammatory compounds into the blood.(22) This helps reduce inflammation and better modulates immune function.

Exercise also corrects and prevents insulin resistance where one fails to properly regulate sugar levels in their blood.(23) Prolonged high blood sugar levels are a major contributor to chronic inflammation.

Exercise improves a person's mental health by stimulating the production of endorphins, the body's natural pain killers and mood elevators. Exercise also reduces the levels of the body's stress hormones, adrenaline and cortisol, which can both contribute to inflammation.(24)

On the other hand, excessive intense exercise, especially in conjunction with inadequate rest, is counterproductive and can worsen inflammation. For example, a study done on athletes who do triathlons revealed signs of low-grade systemic inflammation in those athletes for at least five days after completion of the triathlon.(25) While this inflammation eventually dissipates with adequate rest, athletes who don't take enough recovery time after intense exercise can develop chronic inflammation harming their health.

A number of hypotheses have been proposed to explain this phenomenon. One all-encompassing explanation focuses on the role of pro-inflammatory cytokines in initiating and perpetrating chronic inflammation. The cytokine hypothesis suggests that exercise-induced muscle and connective tissue micro-trauma triggers the release of pro-inflammatory cytokines, which when sufficient rest is allowed, can aid in the healing process. The acute inflammation that results from excessive exercise with inadequate rest on the other hand, evolves into a chronic response resulting in a systemic-wide immune response that involves other organs including the liver and the central nervous system as well as the immune system.(26) Indeed many elite athletes and runners have experienced severe deterioration of their health after years of heavy exercise.

I've always said as with most things in life including exercise, moderation is the key. Regular moderate exercise can include brisk walking for 30 minutes most days. An hour at the swimming pool a few times per week is also a good form of aerobic exercise. And don't forget to do some light weight-bearing exercises to strengthen muscles and help prevent osteoporosis. With this type of regime you will reap all the benefits of exercise without any of the adverse effects of overdoing it.

b. Excessive Stress

When you're overwhelmed by prolonged physical, mental or emotional stress, your adrenal glands release the hormone cortisol. (This stress hormone is released whenever we feel fear, anxiety or worry). Cortisol directly influences your blood sugar levels keeping them consistently elevated and thereby contributing to insulin resistance. (Insulin resistance means that muscle tissue becomes resistant to glucose uptake thereby requiring hyper-secretion of insulin to overcome the muscular resistance). Elevated insulin levels have been shown to have a variety of negative effects upon human metabolism contributing to obesity and low-grade inflammation.

Cortisol is supposed to give us a jolt of energy through its sugar-releasing mechanism enabling us to react to and run away from the perceived danger as it were. However, in this modern world where there are no sabre-tooth tigers to run from but our own psychological stress, then this ongoing stress causes our body systems to be constantly bathed in cortisol.

As well as raising blood sugar levels, cortisol has a secondary function of helping to control the body's inflammatory response. However, when the body is constantly exposed to stress and as a result, cortisol then the body's tissues become less sensitive to cortisol and so release less of their anti-inflammatory compounds. So this means that prolonged stress alters the effectiveness of cortisol to regulate the inflammatory response, thereby in turn, leading to ongoing inflammation that promotes chronic disease.

Prolonged cortisol release has also been associated with thyroid dysfunction which then results in fatigue, weight gain and other problems all of which further compound the effects of inflammation.(27)

c. Lack of Sleep

Making sure you get adequate sleep is important for a number of reasons. We all know that a good night's sleep helps us maintain energy levels to function optimally the next day. It is during sleep that our bodies can best recuperate and regenerate. During sleep the liver purifies the blood while our muscles and tissues repair themselves. In our relaxed sleep state our feel-good neurotransmitters, serotonin and melatonin levels increase. Melatonin is needed to transport sulphate to the brain cells (neurons) at night during sleep. Sulphate, specifically heparin sulphate is required to activate lysosomes, the cell's waste disposal system. However, without adequate sleep (7 to 8 hours per night), insufficient melatonin levels are manufactured in the pineal gland and so, melatonin, being a sulphate delivery system means not enough sulphate in the brain impairs the brain's ability to eliminate heavy metals and other toxins. Melatonin not only transports but also is an outstanding antioxidant that can bind to heavy metals, including cadmium, mercury, lead and aluminium that make their way into the brain, and safely remove these metals from the body.(28)

Sleep is truly the brain's 'housekeeper', the time during which the brain detoxifies by getting rid of cellular debris. Depriving yourself of essential sleep or having interruptive sleep patterns over an extensive period interferes with the brain's detoxification and directly increases the amount of inflammation within the body. Research studies indicate that lack of sleep is directly linked to increased levels of inflammation. Researchers at The University of California, Los Angeles (UCLA) have demonstrated how sleep loss affects the immune system's inflammatory response, causing an overproduction of two pro-inflammatory proteins (fibrinogen and interleukin-B) after a night of sleep loss, compared with amounts found after a night of uninterrupted sleep.

They reported that even modest sleep loss triggers cellular inflammation that can ultimately cause cardiovascular disease, arthritis, diabetes and autoimmune disorders and suggested sleep interventions as a possible way to address problems associated with inflammation.

A 2010 sleep study presented at the American Heart Association Scientific Sessions in Chicago also found a link between raised levels of various pro-inflammatory compounds associated with inadequate sleep. This study which was carried out by scientists at Emory University School of Medicine in Atlanta, found that sleep deprivation or poor sleep quality raises inflammation, which in turn increases the risk of developing heart disease and stroke.(29)

They examined 525 middle-aged people and found that those who get six or fewer hours of sleep each night had twenty five per cent higher levels of the pro-inflammatory C-reactive protein. These individuals also had raised levels of two other pro-inflammatory markers; fibrinogen and interleukin-B.

7. Obesity

It is well known that people who are overweight or obese tend to suffer more of the diseases of ageing. An increasing number of studies show that those with the highest incidence of cardiovascular disease, diabetes, Alzheimer's and depression are invariably overweight.(30) The common link to these health conditions as pointed out in previous parts of this book is ongoing chronic inflammation. This chronic inflammation is also common to obese individuals.

Scientists have now discovered that the inflammation seen in obesity may be caused by body fat. Technically body fat is called 'adipose tissue' and individual fat cells are called adipocytes. Adipocytes consist of about 90% lipids, which are fatty chains bound to a glucose molecule. The other 10% of the cell is composed of water and the mechanisms that govern the cell's functions. Scientists now realise that adipocytes (fat cells) aren't just dormant repositories of excess fat. These fats actually secrete a number of inflammatory mediators including arachidonic acid, which eventually converts into runaway pro-inflammatory compounds such as cytokines and C-reactive proteins.(31)

Further research studies have elicited that the major culprit is central abdominal fat that's involved in the production of these pro-inflammatory compounds. Commonly referred to as "pot belly" or "spare tyre", these fat cells act like small factories in the body to churn out cytokine molecules, which set inflammation in motion. In addition, these fat cells are also storehouses for toxins that could not be safely disposed of due to an over-worked liver. So now, the obese individual gets a double hit of inflammation, on the one hand from their excess fat cells creating inflammation and on the other hand from the stored toxins themselves contributing to more inflammation. We also know that when individuals start to gain weight, their bodies slowly develop a resistance to insulin, whose job is to control blood sugar levels from becoming too high.

To counteract this insulin resistance, the pancreas secrets even more insulin to maintain normal blood sugar levels. Elevated serum insulin levels have been shown to have a variety of negative effects upon human metabolism. For instance, adipose (fat) tissue is highly sensitive to insulin concentration, and a small increase in circulating insulin can greatly elevate fatty acids in the blood. When these fatty acids reach the liver, increased oxidation is stimulated. This event may in and of itself increase the inflammatory response due to unsupported oxygen metabolism, which results in increased levels of lipid peroxidation products and extremely high levels of free radicals.

Studies show that free radicals (unstable oxygen molecules that can cause damage to cell membranes) and lipid peroxidation (the oxidative degradation of lipids by free radicals), strongly stimulates the growth of cancer. To counteract this scenario, I encourage my clients to take a cocktail of antioxidants such as vitamins A, C and E including bioflavonoids, and minerals such as selenium and zinc, which are able to quench the effects of free radicals. Studies show that combinations of multiple antioxidants along with other nutrients that reduce inflammation also reduce the growth and spread of cancer.

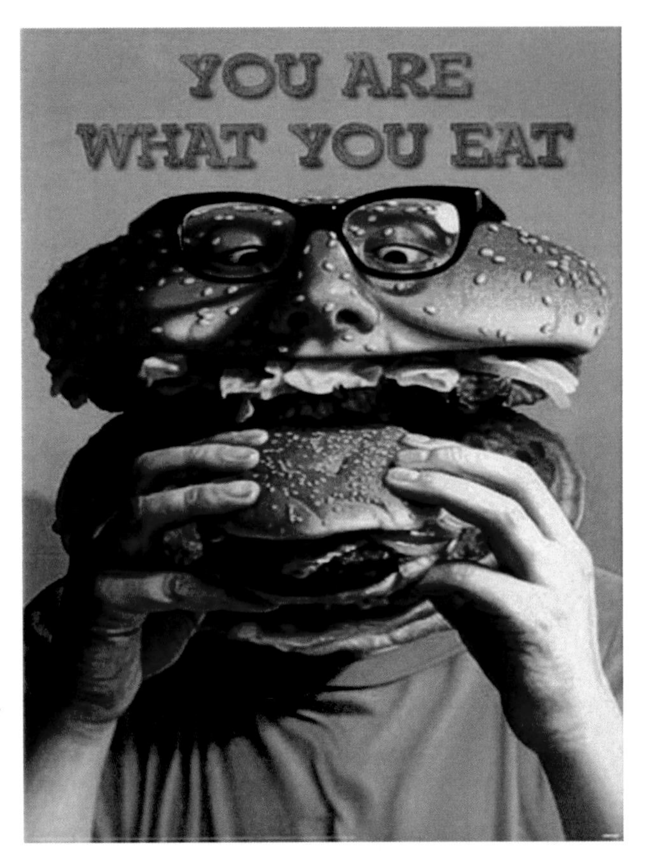

As I previously mentioned, being overweight leads to increased blood serum glucose levels. Tissues that can take up glucose without the mediation of insulin (i.e.: nerves, eyes and kidneys), can end up with excessive glucose concentrations within those tissues. In turn, these tissues promote the formation of advanced glycosylation end products (AGE's), which in turn generates massive amounts of free radicals and lipid peroxidation products causing even more inflammation!

So, the bottom line is, the more fat cells you have, the more inflammation you are creating inside your body, setting the stage for the development of chronic disease and a lifetime of ill health. Therefore, the most important step obese individuals can take is to lose excess weight, which can reduce inflammation in a matter of weeks or months.

A study published in the journal JAMA of Internal Medicine in 2007 which analysed results of 33 separate studies, found that losing weight can lower C-reactive protein (an inflammation marker) levels by 0.13mg per litre of blood for every kilogram (2.2 pounds) of weight loss.(32) So by my calculations if you manage to lose 8kg which is about 1st 3lbs, you will reduce your C-reactive protein levels by 1.0mg/L. According to the American Heart Association, a C-reactive protein level of less than 1.0mg/L indicates a low risk of cardiovascular disease while above 3.0mg/L is high risk.

Do you want to start losing flab very quickly?

You don't have to count calories or follow some complicated diet plan; all you have to do is cut out these 3 foods from your diet for the next few weeks:

1. Processed foods. If it comes in a box or a package with a laundry list of ingredients, eliminate it. Instead, concentrate on eating mostly whole, natural foods.

2. Soft drinks, fruit juices, and other sweetened beverages. Drinks sweetened with sugar actually *increase* your hunger while feeding you loads of empty calories.

3. Alcohol. Alcohol is calorie dense and further wreaks havoc on your fat burning hormones, increasing your belly fat and making it harder for you to lose that spare tyre.

Want to get a flat belly fast?

Simply follow the above 3 rules. You will automatically eliminate a *massive* amount of calories from your diet and you'll still be able to eat until you're full, while achieving rapid results. *Put them in place today!*

8. Injury

It sounds like stating the obvious when I say that injury to body cells and tissues cause inflammation. But when the injury is not properly resolved, then it can progress to chronic inflammation.

When I'm talking about injury in this context, I'm referring to cellular and tissue injury that can result from a number of circumstances. Infection is one example; other causes include physical trauma as in blunt impact with another object, or cuts and bruises, or exposure to excessive heat or extreme cold. Injury also results from both external and internal toxin contact and also from allergic reactions.

Whatever the underlying factor that causes injury, the immune system is immediately activated and releases a variety of biological mediators to trigger an acute inflammatory response that serves as a mechanism initiating the elimination of any noxious agents and repairing damaged tissues. When the source of the injury is eliminated by this powerful process, the immune system response ceases and inflammation stops ideally. However, if the inflammatory process is unchecked or if the inflammation is unresolved due to the source of the injury persisting, then this acute inflammatory process leads to the development of ongoing chronic inflammation.

For instance, injuries occurring especially among older people can invariably lead to chronic inflammation as a result of the natural decline in the cell renewal process. As we age, the structure of our tissue changes and as our cells die off, the resultant void is increasingly filled with collagen fibres, producing scar tissue. Any repeated damage to imperfectly repaired tissues can contribute to more generalized inflammation.

Another example may be when an individual suffers ongoing back pain due to a damaged disc. Because of the physiological nature of this type of injury, the injured disc can suffer repeated injury during the active healing phase leading to persistent inflammation, resulting in enhanced disc degeneration.

9. Low-Grade Metabolic Acidosis

According to Professor Enderlein (a renowned German biologist 1872-1968) ***"there is only one sickness and that is the over-acidification of the blood and tissues caused by an inverted way of eating and living".***

In this one sentence he has summarized most of what I've already portrayed as the causative factors of inflammation. In essence he is stating that when one's body becomes overly acidic (a condition known as "low-grade metabolic acidosis"), this condition jeopardizes the optimal functioning of the body, thereby leaving the host vulnerable to disease.

Many healthcare researchers and health practitioners agree that an over-acidic body is connected in most part with poor diet and lifestyle. For instance, during the normal process of metabolism, the body will convert food into energy. This process will create different acids along with the acids already present in the food source. This will increase the acid levels in our body and if these acids are not neutralized and eliminated through our kidneys, lungs and bowels, then the body's acid-alkaline balance weighs heavily towards the acidic side and the end result is metabolic acidosis.

I'd like to make a clear distinction here, between the term "low-grade metabolic acidosis", which is what I'll be talking about in this section and the more extreme forms of acidosis that doctors would be familiar with – these include:

- **Keto-acidosis** that occurs when diabetics start burning their own fat;
- **Renal-acidosis**, which is sign of kidney failure; and
- **Lactic-acidosis** from over-exercise and/or oxygen deficiency.

These conditions are all life -threatening and require immediate life-saving help.

Low-grade metabolic acidosis on the other hand is caused by a persistent build-up of excess metabolic acids within the body. Rather than causing immediate symptoms as in the more extreme acute forms of acidosis, this low-grade acidosis, over time, becomes chronic leading to a host of health problems that are often attributed to other causes such as ageing or calcium deficiencies.

So, maintaining a normal acid-alkaline balance within the body is one of the most important parameters of health. And according to many health researchers and practitioners alike, true healing of any health condition can only take place when the blood and body tissues are first restored to a slightly alkaline state.

If you've forgotten your high school chemistry class, then allow me to refresh it:- the body's acid-alkaline balance is measured on the pH scale ranging from 0 to 14. pH stands for "potential of hydrogen". This means that the relative concentration of hydrogen ions influences acid-alkaline balance. Pure water (H_2O) has a pH of 7 which is neutral. A pH below 7 is acidic while pH above 7 is alkaline. Stomach acid (HCL) has a pH of around 2.5, while household bleach (ammonia) has a pH of 11.5.

A slight change in pH corresponds to a strong modification of the hydrogen ion concentration, which is ten times higher from one number to another. For instance:

pH 7 = neutral (pure H2O, water)

pH 6 = 10 times more acidic

pH 5 = 10 x 10 = 100 times more acidic

The ideal body pH is 7.0 or slightly alkaline at 7.1. Human blood pH should always remain slightly alkaline in the range 7.35 – 7.45. Deviations above or below this range can signal potentially serious health conditions. In fact, our bodies will go to great lengths to maintain a blood pH of 7.35 that it will create stress on other tissues, organs and body systems to do so. This in turn will lead to acidic wastes accumulating in cells and tissue spaces interrupting normal cellular function.

Our body tissues and the fluids between our cells tend to be slightly acidic with an average pH of 6.9. This is because by nature the body is acid producing, however it functions better in a slightly alkaline state. Under normal conditions, the body constantly regulates acidity through numerous biochemical processes to buffer and remove acids from the body. However, if these pH buffering systems becomes depleted or can't cope due to the constant build-up of excess metabolic acids in the body, then this tilt towards greater acidity produces a fertile breeding ground for a variety of health problems including muscle weakness, heart disease, diabetes, osteoporosis, kidney problems and more.

There are many factors that can influence your body's pH. Nutrition, lifestyle choices and even mental attitudes like psychological stress and anxiety can create acidity within the body tissues. Other factors include alkaline-mineral deficiencies, lack of or excess physical exercise, inadequate breathing or any process that deprives the cells of oxygen and dehydration. Also included are things like allergies, toxins and immune reactions.

But chief among them is your diet. The typical modern-day diet is far too high in acid-producing animal products like meat, dairy and eggs and far too low in alkaline-producing foods like fresh vegetables, fruits and salads. Additionally, we eat acid-producing processed foods like white flour and high sugar content foods. We drink acid-producing beverages such as tea and coffee, alcohol and soft drinks. Additionally, substances added to our foods such as artificial sweeteners along with the thousands of other chemical additives are also extremely acid-forming.

By consistently eating too many acid-forming foods and not balancing the equation by eating more alkaline-producing foods, we will eventually end up suffering from chronic low-grade metabolic acidosis.

A major consequence of this over-acidity of body tissues is inflammation. Think of the corrosive nature of acids and then imagine what happens to your tissues and organs as more and more acid wastes build up, leaving your body to stew in its poisonous wastes. A chronically over-acidic body pH will corrode body tissues, increasing the release of inflammatory free radicals making inflammation and pain even worse. Also, when the body's pH becomes acidic, oxygen delivery to cells decreases. This then results in anaerobic respiration (without oxygen) within the cells that produces even more acidic waste by-products (i.e. lactic acid) causing further inflammation. In addition, an acidic environment is also a fertile ground for the proliferation of harmful micro-organisms, which again contributes to more inflammation.

So when the body tissues and organs are chronically exposed to acidosis the resultant corrosion and inflammation causes these tissues to harden, swell and develop lesions in order to protect themselves. If the inflammation persists, and it will as long as the acidic condition remains, then it will eventually lead to a variety of disease conditions such as arthritis, osteoporosis, skin diseases, accelerated ageing, digestive disorders, chronic infections, cancer, diabetes, heart disease, and so on. In fact, when our pH is unbalanced long-term, the end result is a multitude of chronic conditions. So if you don't feel good, one of the basic things that stands between you and perfect health is your body's pH.

It is primarily the kidneys job to balance the body's acid-alkaline balance by co-ordinating a number of buffering systems to neutralize excess acid build up. These buffering systems need a good balance of alkalizing minerals to work effectively. If we are not getting an adequate amount of these minerals from our diet, then our body will start borrowing these minerals from our bones and tissues. Our bones will release calcium and magnesium while our muscles are broken down to release ammonia. The long term consequences of allowing this process to continue unabated are thinner bones and lower muscle mass. Calcium and magnesium are essential for healthy bone formation and also for normal heart function. Low magnesium levels can also result in abnormal heart arrhythmias, muscle cramps and anxiety states.

How many times have you heard of, or read in the papers about some middle-aged executive who without proper training decides to run in some charity race like a mini-marathon, only to fall down dead with a heart attack. Their acidity levels were already extremely high due to their diet and stressful lifestyle and work environment before commencing their run. No doubt their calcium and magnesium reserves were also bordering at dangerously low levels, which could precipitate a potentially lethal heart arrhythmia. All that was needed then to tip them over the edge was a sudden surge in lactic acid brought about by over exertion!

Now, when the kidneys ability to neutralize and eliminate this acid build up is overloaded, then the body suffers from low-grade metabolic acidosis. Some of the early symptomatologies we start to experience are low energy levels, poor digestion and bloating. We may begin to gain weight as a protective measure to help store away excess acids in our fat cells. Our thinking becomes unclear; and we can begin to experience anxiety and depression. We may begin to suffer from niggling aches and pains; in fact you cannot have pain without acid or acidity without pain. Acids affect our nervous system, our muscles become tenderised and begin to break down, our skin tone deteriorates, ageing and wrinkling start to surface, our brain becomes foggy and our organs become weak and overall we just feel sick and tired!!

Tips for a balanced pH

Eating to maintain a slightly alkaline pH is easier than you might think as a pH-friendly diet is consistent with other healthy eating habits. When my clients start eating a more alkaline diet, their main health problems diminish along with their many other niggling problems such as low energy levels, aches and pains, skin rashes, catarrhal problems, headaches and so on. Here's what I recommend:

- The simplest way to increase alkaline foods in the diet is to increase the amount of fresh fruit and vegetables in the diet and to cut down on acid-producing foods such as animal products, sugar and acid-forming beverages (see the list of Acid/Alkaline Forming Foods in Appendix 5). Generally alkaline forming foods include most fruits, green vegetables (especially dark leafy greens), salads, nuts and seeds, herbs and spices.
- Generally acid-forming foods include all animal products including red and white meats, dairy, eggs, grains (including wheat, barley and oats), caffeinated beverages, alcohol, sugar, processed foods and legumes. Go easy on these foods.
- Stay hydrated: that means drinking more water, not tea, coffee, soft drinks or alcohol, which serves only to dehydrate the body even more. As a general rule, you should drink forty millilitres of water for every kilogram of body weight. So a 70kg person should consume 70 x 40ml = 2.8 litres of water daily. A squeeze of lemon in our water adds taste and has an alkalizing effect in your body.
- Drinks which feature ingredients such as wheatgrass, barley grass, spiralina and chlorella are all very alkalizing. These green super foods usually come as powders and can be mixed in a glass of water. Fresh vegetable juices are also excellent to drink and can include vegetables such as carrots, celery, spinach, cabbage, parsley and any other green vegetables.

- Remove salt from the table or if you must use it, then opt for sea salt as it has a range of alkalizing minerals. Regular salt consists of sodium and chloride, both of which contribute to acidosis.
- Managing stress helps keep your body healthy. When you stress, cortisol (a stress hormone) levels will rise, which can contribute to increased acidity.
- Taking supplements such as calcium and magnesium to help neutralize metabolic acidosis. Both minerals are alkaline and offer a substantial contribution to keeping the body's pH balanced. Opt for the citrate form as in calcium citrate and magnesium citrate as these forms are easily absorbed and metabolized to bicarbonates that act as systemic alkalinizers. Fumarate, aspartate and succinate forms of minerals also have an alkalizing effect.

To summarise:

It's important to remember that acid-forming foods are not bad per se and therefore are needed as part of a balanced diet. The key is to eat sufficient alkaline-forming foods to offset acid-forming foods. For example, a ham and cheese sandwich is entirely acid-forming on its own, but can be balanced with the addition of salads or an avocado. A steak for dinner needs to be balanced with plenty of vegetables. Breakfast cereal with cow's milk (all acid), can be balanced with some chopped fruit and so on.

Summary of the causes of Inflammation

To recap what you read in this chapter regarding the underlying causes of how inflammation starts and continues in the body. Here's a brief summary:-

- ➢ Too much fat consumption, especially hydrogenated fats and imbalanced omega-6 to omega-3 fat intake, sugar, processed and fast foods as well as over-proportioned amounts of dairy products and red meats.
- ➢ Persistent chronic low-grade infections resulting from a range of micro-organisms as diverse as viruses, bacteria, fungi and parasites. The by-products of these organisms are toxic to body tissues thereby causing inflammation
- ➢ Environmental toxins from air, water and soil including pesticides,

herbicides, fungicides, pollution, heavy metals, chemicals in foods and personal care products and most man-made chemicals.

- An imbalance of micro flora in your digestive tract leading to increased levels of endogenous toxins that among other things can cause a leaky gut.
- Imbalanced eating especially diets high in animal products that cause an imbalance in metabolism, resulting in toxins being produced within the body.
- Dehydration caused by lack of water intake, excessive sweating, diarrhoea, excessive urination or by drinking too much caffeinated beverages.
- Food allergy and food intolerances.
- Lifestyle factors such as:
  - Lack of exercise or excessive exercise such a marathon running, can both contribute to inflammation.
  - High psychological stress-levels increase the hormone cortisol, which over time fuels inflammation.
  - Lack of sleep and sleep problems whether caused by emotional or medical reasons raises inflammation due to an inability of the body to properly recuperate from the previous day's stresses.
- Obesity: the fatty tissues of the body secrete hormones that regulate the immune system and promote inflammation. The more fat cells one has, the more the immune system is provoked into an inflammatory mode.
- Injuries that do not heal properly or are repeatedly being traumatized.
- pH balance: the over acidification of the blood and tissues caused by one or all of the above factors or as in the words of Enderlein, "due to an inverted way of eating and living".

So what can we do to resolve these underlying causes of inflammation that leads to ill health? Read on…….

CHAPTER 3

TAKING BACK CHARGE OF YOUR HEALTH

> *"The doctor of the future will give no medicine, but will interest his patient in the care of the human frame, in diet and in the cause and prevention of disease" –*
> *Thomas Edison*

The most profound insight I ever gleaned about staying healthy came to me after years of witnessing truly remarkable recoveries of the many clients who frequented my health centre. In a nutshell it is this: - our marvellous human body possesses the incredible ability to detoxify, repair and renew itself for as long as we live. In fact your body is performing this near miraculous feat this very moment as you read this. No matter how old you are, your body will generate new skin, bone tissue and muscle cells. Your immune system will continue to fight and conquer micro-organisms and your injuries and bruises will heal just like they always have. There's just one catch: you must provide your body's remarkable healing and repair power with the correct

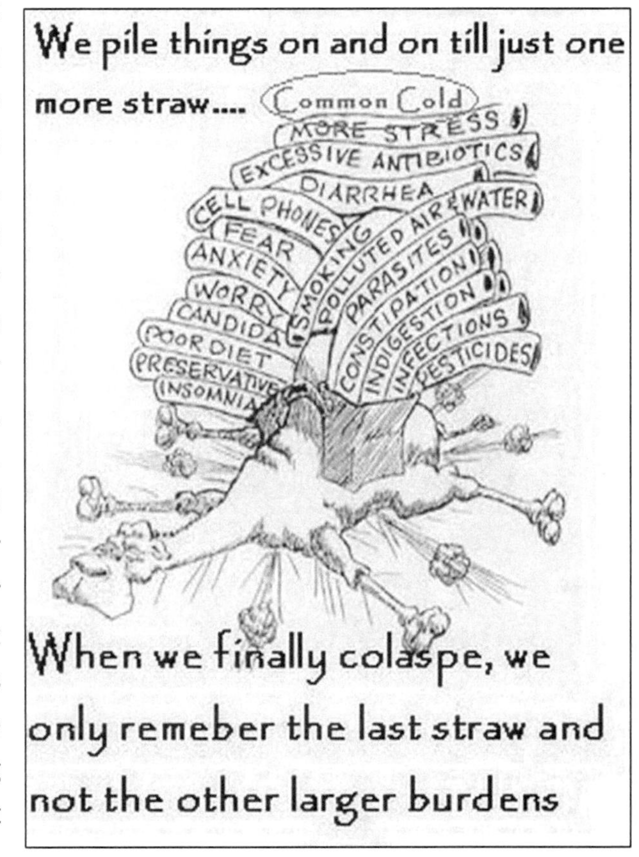

nutritional materials and building blocks it needs to keep going and growing.

There are a number of very simple, clear and inexpensive steps that we can all take to improve our health status. Good health and vibrant well-being is the normal state for the human body and under natural conditions should continue from birth until the grave, hopefully at a very old age. So disease conditions like arthritis, heart disease, obesity, digestive disorders, skin disease, autoimmune diseases, along with a host of other disorders rarely arise because of defects in the body, they occur because we unwittingly make them happen through our erroneous choices.

As previously explained in this book most, if not all of the underlying causes of ill health can be summed up in our inverted way of everyday living. Our modern diet and toxic environment coupled with daily stresses and lack of exercise are some of the key areas we need to contend with. The state of your body; how it looks and feels as well as how it functions depends to an enormous extent on how well it is nourished; along with its ability to detoxify. The unavoidable toxins of modern life – in the water you drink, the air you breathe and the food you eat, are building up in your body and destroying your health, increasing your risk of chronic and fatal diseases.

Medical science has shown that the accumulation of these toxins leads to immune system dysfunction resulting in chronic ongoing inflammation, which results in fatigue, premature ageing, degenerative conditions, etc, etc. Our body is constantly endeavouring to detoxify itself, but if it becomes overloaded with toxins and impurities it will eventually malfunction and shut down.

Just how critical is it to get rid of toxins in your body? Well, Dr. J. H. Tilden, author of "Toxaemia Explained" makes the admonition that *"All sickness, all disease and all death is caused by the progressive accumulation of toxaemia (poison) in the body and the blood".*(33)

It stands to reason then, that an individual's health is largely determined by their ability to detoxify. Deciding whether or not to support your body's detoxification system is like choosing whether you want your body to be a pristine clean and healthy ecosystem, or a pathogenic infested and toxic waste dump! The answer is obvious, of course you want to flush out toxic poisons and pathogenic micro-organisms and regain optimal health in the process.

In this and the following chapters I'll show you measures you can take to safely detoxify your body, starting first with the gastro-intestinal tract, then focussing on the liver, blood and kidneys and finishing with the skin, lungs and lymphatic system. I also devote a separate chapter to support for the nervous system, as no other body systems can function effectively when the nervous system is in any way compromised.

Herxheimer Reaction

A word of warning about a phenomenon you may experience when embarking upon a natural detox programme. As your body detoxifies you may start experiencing a worsening of symptoms lasting from a couple of days to a few weeks duration.

Although uncomfortable, this is just a short-term reaction in the body, otherwise known as the "Herxheimer Reaction". The term was coined to describe what Karl Herxheimer, a German dermatologist saw when he administered drugs to his patients.

The reaction is believed to happen when released endotoxins from dead pathogens (viruses, bacteria, candida, parasites) overwhelm the body's abilities to clear them out. This results in a toxic state being created in the body, which produces flu-like symptoms including headaches, joint and muscle pain, general malaise, chills and fevers, skin eruptions (acne, hives, rashes), excess mucus production, nausea and diarrhoea, or other symptoms.

The more endotoxins that are present in the body, the stronger the Herxheimer reaction will be.The biggest problem with the Herxheimer reaction is that people stop taking their medication or quit the detox process before completion, in the misguided belief that the treatment is not working but instead causing an allergic reaction. Although the worsening symptoms may be somewhat uncomfortable, they do not indicate failure of the treatment in question – in fact, the Herxheimer reaction is actually a sign that healing is taking place.

Ways to Ameliorate the Herxheimer Reaction

- Drink plenty of filtered water to help flush out the toxins faster. You can also add some lemon juice, which stimulates the liver.
- Reduce the dosage of your medication (e.g. Herbal tonic) to slow down the detoxification process.
- Take activated charcoal which helps absorb toxins from the bowel.
- Take extra vitamin C and E.
- Increase sweating via an infrared sauna, which is an excellent way to remove heavy metals, pesticides and other toxic chemicals from the body.
- Have Epsom salts baths, which also pulls out toxins via the skin. A floatation tank (see page 112) filled with 400kg of Epsom salts, is an amazing way to detoxify while the body remains in a deeply relaxed state.
- Massage helps to release toxins that have solidified inside muscles.
- Make sure you get plenty of rest and sleep. Your body needs energy to dispel toxins. The more you rest the quicker your body can detoxify.

The Gastrointestinal Detox and Repair Programme

The digestive system is the most important place to start detoxification. There is an old naturopathic saying that **"death begins in the colon".** It may sound clichéd but it still holds true; you see our colon is a sewage system that when abused and neglected can, over time, become a toxic cesspool. When it is clean and functioning normal we are well and happy, let it stagnate and it will distil the poisons of decay, fermentation and putrefaction into the blood and tissues causing auto-intoxication of every organ of the body, leading us to age prematurely and suffer from a myriad of chronic diseases with the consequent pleasure-of-living being gone.

To reverse this condition requires a bowel cleansing and repair program designed to correct gut dysbiosis (abnormal amounts of pathogenic bacteria, yeasts and parasite infestation in the bowel). Once the bowel is clean and free of pathogens and their toxic by-products, then we can focus on repairing the gut wall and re-colonizing the colon with friendly bacteria. By healing the bowel wall, toxins are prevented from leaking through it into the bloodstream.

The best method I have found when it comes to cleaning, repairing and optimizing gastrointestinal function is through a program pioneered by the health scientists at the Institute of Functional Medicine called the **four R's** of gut health.(34) The four R's stand for:

- **Remove**
- **Repair**
- **Replace**
- **Re-inoculate**

Remove

The first step to restoring healthy gastrointestinal function is to reduce exposure to reactive foods and environmental toxins. There are tonnes of toxins that can trigger inflammation and food is one of them. You must watch what you eat. The modern diet of processed foods high in sugars and low in fibre produce a kind of sludge within the gastrointestinal system that clogs up the bowel. This build-up of old, rotting food and waste is the perfect breeding ground for all kinds of harmful micro-organisms.

It's toxic and acidic properties irritates and inflames the colon walls causing a leaky gut wall, allowing toxins, bacteria, chemicals and undigested food particles to enter the bloodstream, where they can cause inflammation and dysfunction in many organs and tissues.

Studies reveal most colons are plugged up with old rotting waste material. The most famous colon study was carried out by German doctor Arnold Ehret, the legendary expert on colons and colon autopsies. He examined the colons of 284 deceased people and was stunned to discover that out of 284 autopsies only 28 colons were found to be free from hardened faeces. The others contained hardened, rotten faecal material.(35)

Other colon studies have shown that even people who defecate once daily can still have faecal impaction in their colons. This is referred to as hidden constipation and this putrid build-up can remain undetected for a lifetime.

I've had many clients who for years have a bowel motion less than once daily and sometimes only twice a week. Many of them had been informed by their well-meaning physicians that having bowel movements twice a week is sufficient. This is very bad advice. The bowel accumulates a great number of toxins and without regular elimination they will be re-circulated into the bloodstream. People should have at least one bowel movement every day and preferably one after each meal.

Getting your colon back in regular working order is the number one thing you can do to help restore and protect your health. The truth is you can't be healthy if your colon is sick! At my health centre I stock a colon cleanser called "Oxy FX" which does a superb job of removing years of impacted food matter and putrid faeces lodged in your colon. More information on Oxy FX can be found in the inserted box on page 66.

Getting back to your diet, you'll need to remove problematic foods you may be intolerant of or allergic to. Utilizing an elimination diet is the best way to pinpoint whether you are reacting to foods. While it takes between one and three months to follow the steps outlined in the elimination diet (See Appendix 4), you will be able to determine what foods might be responsible for a lot of your symptoms. Once you have eliminated these foods from your diet, you may be able to maintain your symptom-free status long term.

The successful treatment of gut dysbiosis requires correct food choices and much persistence on your behalf. If you are not willing to give up problematic foods, then you will most likely not have any relief in symptoms no matter how many supplements or prescriptions you take. Removing these foods is the quickest route to regaining a healthy gut and reclaiming optimal health.

To achieve a successful outcome you may require the services of a natural health practitioner to help you with these dietary changes and where appropriate, suggest supplements and other natural products to assist in a bowel cleansing and repair program.

It's also imperative to remove from the gastrointestinal tract any disease causing micro-organisms, including pathogenic bacteria, fungi and parasites, which all cause inflammation and damage to the intestinal mucosa.

Many health therapists treat their clients based upon the assumption that there is a yeast (candida) overgrowth or a parasite present, etc. I do not like making this assumption. The way I figure it, if you're going to be treated for candida overgrowth or parasites, it's best to figure out exactly what you should be eliminating. After all, just as antibiotics or anti-fungals work differently in the body, so too do various herbal and nutritional substances. Whether or not you have pathogenic organisms or parasites in your gut can be determined by specialist diagnostic tests that I utilize at my health centre. You can read more about these tests in Chapter 11.

Depending on what these tests reveal I may prescribe herbal formulae that can include herbs like Pau D'arco and Oregon grape which are effective in reducing the numbers of unfriendly bacteria and yeast spores. Nutrients such as zinc and biotin may also be recommended as they assist in fungal control while also helping to heal damaged intestinal mucosa.

Oxy FX

Of all the chemical elements, oxygen is the most vital to the human body. We would survive for only a few minutes without oxygen. The only way to truly optimise health is to ensure complete cellular oxygenation. Every one of the body's fifty trillion cells demands oxygen for proper function. Oxygen starvation at cellular level (hypoxia) is the underlying cause of most diseases.

Oxy FX is a combination of powdered magnesium oxide compounds, which have been ozonated and stabilized to release pure oxygen over a 12 hour period. The timed release ensures that Oxy FX will provide an adequate amount of oxygen, slowly, for better utilization.

Many of us suffer from varying degrees of toxaemia and low oxygen levels, due to our diet and lifestyle choices. This results in insufficient metabolism causing the body to accumulate waste products faster than it can eliminate them. Pathogens proliferate in an oxygen poor environment. Because pathogens are essentially anaerobic, they cannot survive and will die when ideal oxygen levels are once again achieved.

Oxy FX when ingested begins to slowly release pure oxygen into the digestive system. This begins to immediately soften intestinal plaque and hardened faeces, kill pathogenic microbes and purify and energise intestinal cells. As the now liquefied plaque and faecal waste along with dead pathogens are ready to be eliminated from the body the magnesium component creates a colon flushing reaction that increases bowel activity and prevents re-absorption of the toxins.

Oxy FX accomplishes a very thorough inner cleanse with none of the risks of customary colonics or enemas, and the cleansing effect reaches the entire digestive tract.

I also find intestinal parasites can be a major problem for a lot of my clients. Parasites can cause extensive damage to the gut wall and are difficult to eliminate. Fortunately, I stock safe and effective herbs that can kill and eliminate potentially dangerous parasites and their eggs from the bowel. Examples include wormwood, black walnut, cloves, tansy, garlic and grapefruit seed extract.

In dealing with conditions like constipation, I would formulate a blend of natural herbal ingredients designed to loosen and remove deeply impacted toxic build-up in the colon, while the oxygen-rich cleansing supplement called "Oxy FX" will naturally push this debris out of your bowels each morning.

Also, during the "remove phase" of the 4 R program, other things to avoid include the use of antibiotics, antacids and anti-inflammatory drugs.

And finally, mental stress and negative emotional states can also have devastating effects on your digestive system (more about this in chapter 9) and so should not be overlooked. So be mindful of this by taking the time to relax and rest and only eat when you're in a calm state.

In summary:

The main purpose of the "remove phase" is to reduce inflammation of the gut mucosa. Much of what has been suggested in this phase should be ongoing and can be ongoing indefinitely.

Repair

The next step is to begin to repair the gut by healing the damaged intestinal mucosa. Over time the lining of the intestinal tract becomes damaged due to all the irritants and stressors mentioned in Step 1. An injured intestinal lining can become 'leaky' allowing partially digested food particles, pathogenic organisms along with other toxins and chemicals to be absorbed into the bloodstream. As you are now aware, these substances will be recognized as foreign invaders to the body and can end up triggering an immune response causing inflammation, which can manifest as a myriad of symptoms throughout the body.

Luckily, the lining of the gut is constantly renewing itself and so, can be repaired fairly easily given the right conditions. In fact the full lining of the gastrointestinal tract is completely replaced about once a week. So with this in mind we know that intestinal cells have a very high metabolic demand (need for nutrients) in order to carry out their functions properly as well as divide so rapidly.

So, in order to return your intestines to their healthy well-functioning state they need to be supplied with all the essential nutrients they require to heal and aid repair of the mucosal cells. Certainly, part of the support for healing comes from first removing the stressor foods, toxins and pathogens that continually re-injure and irritate the intestinal mucosa.

The following nutrients will help significantly in the repair of the intestinal tract lining:

- **L-Glutamine:** This is an amino acid that is the preferred food source for the cells of the gastrointestinal mucosa. It helps to heal and rebuild the lining of the intestinal tract. L-Glutamine is also part of the compound glutathione which provides additional protection from inflammation to help in healing. L-Glutamine comes in capsules or as a powder that you should take first thing in the morning and at night before bed.
- **Aloe Vera:** This mucilaginous plant has long been used internally for its laxative and cleansing properties. It is soothing to all tissues and has remarkable healing powers on the gut lining. One should begin aloe therapy at a dosage of one teaspoonful daily and work up to a suitable dosage of around one tablespoonful one to two times daily.
- **Liquorice Root:** This herb is an effective treatment for any gastrointestinal inflammations due to its superior tissue healing properties. Liquorice has been proven to be among the best anti-ulcer medications available and one that I regularly use as part of my herbal formulae for repairing damaged mucosal linings.
- **Multivitamin and Mineral Formulae:** Correction of nutritional deficiencies especially vitamins A, B9, B12 and the mineral zinc are required for intestinal cells to repair efficiently. These nutrients also assist in the detoxification of

many chemicals by the gut and liver cells. Every adult irrespective of age should take a daily multivitamin and multimineral supplement to help offset any underlying nutrient deficiency that invariably occurs due to bad dietary choices, lifestyle factors and disease processes.

- **Omega 3 fatty acids and their derivatives gamma linoleic acid (GLA) and docosahexaenoic acid (DHA).** Found predominantly in fish oil, these compounds are particularly effective in reducing inflammation in the gastrointestinal tract and also are part of the structure of the mucosal cell membranes. They also play an important role in the body's immune system. They are abundant in cold water fish such as mackerel, herring, tuna, salmon and sardines, and can also be taken as a supplement.

In summary:

The main purpose of the "repair phase" is to re-establish good digestive function once inflammation has been reduced or eliminated.

Replace

This stage is where we continue to focus on restoring digestive function by getting the body's digestive enzymes, stomach acid (HCL) and bile salts to optimal levels to maintain and promote healthy digestion. In order to digest our food fully we need sufficient amounts of hydrochloric acid (HCL), the full range of digestive enzymes and bile acids from the liver, all of which tend to be compromised by dietary indiscretions, medications, nutrient deficiencies, ageing and ill health. If any of these digestive substances are at insufficient levels, food will only be partially digested and this will manifest as a sense of fullness after eating. Also, symptoms like bloating, belching, flatulence, heartburn and constipation or diarrhoea are other common indicators of incomplete digestion.

When it comes to improving digestion one needs to first learn to chew their food properly. Chewing not only breaks food into smaller pieces, it also mixes it with the digestive enzymes in the saliva and signals to the digestive system that food is coming.

To break down foods more efficiently some of the following recommendations can be tried 15-20 minutes before each meal:

- Paw-paw eaten 15-20 minutes before a meal will provide digestive enzymes to promote digestion of that meal. Lemon juice sprinkled on top will disguise the odour that many find objectionable.
- Pineapples also contain digestive enzymes. They can be eaten before meals or the core can be soaked overnight in water and left in the fridge. A few tablespoonfuls of the water will contain enough enzymes to help digest a meal the next day. This water can also be placed in a small bottle to sip on before a meal if eating out at a restaurant.
- Alfalfa seeds. One tablespoonful soaked overnight in a small glass of water will contain enough enzymes to break down proteins taken in the diet. This water can also be placed in a small bottle to sip on if out for lunch or dinner. It works really well for all ages, but is particularly effective in young children and babies suffering from a lot of mucus congestion, running noses and glue ear.
- You can also supplement with store bought digestive enzymes. Typical brands will usually contain a variety of enzymes such as amylase, lipase, pepsin, lactase and trypsin. Some brands may also contain hydrochloric acid to improve stomach acidity.
- Another digestive factor that often needs enhancement is the stomach's hydrochloric acid levels. People who suffer from indigestion, belching or heartburn are usually low in hydrochloric acid! – often mistaken for too much stomach acid. As people age, they naturally produce less HCL and gastric juices.

Ways to increase stomach acid include:

- Apple cider vinegar: One tablespoonful placed in a cup of hot water with one teaspoon of honey to taste, will stimulate the stomach's digestive processes into action. Take 15 minutes before eating.

- Lemon juice in water will also stimulate the digestive processes of the stomach.
- Hydrochloric acid production depends on zinc, so be aware that low stomach acid may indicate a zinc deficiency. Other zinc deficiency signs to look out for include white spots on the nails, loss of smell and taste, delayed wound healing, stretch marks or lack of dream recall.
- Other considerations to help improve digestion include not drinking a lot of fluids with meals as this tends to dilute digestive juices and enzymes.
- Eating smaller meals puts less of a burden on your digestive system. Also, eat more raw foods as they already come pre-packaged with the enzymes needed to break them down. Cooking destroys these enzymes.

In summary:

The main purpose of the "replace phase" is to assist the digestive system to convert the food you eat into vitamins, minerals, amino acids and other nutrients so your body can easily absorb them.

Re-inoculate

This step involves the restoration of your gut's friendly bacteria population. You carry about 100 trillion bacteria in your gut whose weight is approximately 1 kg. You may be surprised to know that these bacteria outnumber your body cells by a ratio of about 2:1. In a healthy gut, there should be a ratio of about 80:20 good bacteria to bad bacteria but circumstance such as bad diet, overuse of antibiotics and other medications including the contraceptive pill, along with various other factors skew the percentage the other way in favour of bad bacteria. This situation allows for gut health to drastically decline.

In a normal healthy intestine, the friendly bacteria produce molecules called short chain fatty acids that are used directly to nourish the mucosal cells lining the intestinal walls. With the loss of these beneficial bacteria the intestinal cells literally starve to death. Compounding the problem then is the opportunistic overgrowth of the bad bacteria, fungi and other microorganisms that cause inflammation and damage to the gastrointestinal mucosa.

Researchers who study the gut bacteria have identified over 500 different strains of bacteria.(36) These researchers often refer to these bacteria as the 'microbial organ', due to the fact that these microorganisms perform a host of useful functions beneficial to the body. For instance, these good bacteria synthesize vitamins such as biotin and vitamin K; they produce fuel for mucosal cells; metabolise and safely degrades toxins, bile acids and hormones present in the digestive tract, and prevent the overgrowth of harmful pathogenic bacteria.

In order to promote healthy intestine flora, we need to replenish the gut with supplemental **probiotics** and **prebiotics.**

Probiotics consists of friendly bacteria with various strains such as Lactobacillus acidophilus and Bifido bacteria that are capable of restoring the protective bacterial populations, while also reducing the harmful bacteria levels. Probably the most important role probiotics play is in keeping dangerous microorganisms at bay.

Prebiotics are the foods that these friendly bacteria eat in order to flourish. Fructo-oligosaccharides (FOS) is a prebiotic fibre that your body cannot digest, but is a good food source for the friendly bacteria. Some probiotic brands include it as part of their formula, but it can also be taken separately as a powder.

Both probiotics and prebiotics can also be taken in the form of fermented foods such as natural yoghurt, miso, kefir and sauerkraut.

In summary:

The main purpose of the "Re-inoculate Phase" is to control and minimise dangerous microorganisms by replenishing the intestines with friendly bacteria, whose functions also include detoxification, immune system support, micronutrient synthesis, hormone balancing and nutrition for the body's cells.

If you follow the 4R Program diligently for a period of three to six months, you will no doubt succeed in fully restoring gastrointestinal function to optimal levels. And remember, creating a healthy gastrointestinal tract is the key to ALL other systems functioning efficiently in the body.

CHAPTER 4

LIVER DETOXIFICATION

> ***"Disease doesn't just happen overnight. Heart disease, cancers, - most ALL diseases - develop months, even years after your liver failed to keep your blood clean"***
>
> ***- Dr. Richard Schulze***

The liver is one of the most important organs in the body when it comes to detoxifying. It is a large three to five pound organ that sits under your right rib cage. Unlike most organs with just a handful of jobs to perform, your liver performs over five hundred different functions including detoxification of the body. The liver can even regenerate its own tissue. For instance, if 90% of your liver was removed, the remaining 10% could regenerate into a complete organ!

It operates like a massive chemical plant, manufacturing certain compounds, detoxifying dangerous chemicals and directing substances all over the body either for use, storage or excretion.

Its functions can be divided into three basic areas:

1) **Vascular:**

   The liver is a major blood reservoir, filtering almost 1½ litres of blood per minute for detoxification. During filtration, the liver breaks down and removes any substances toxic to our bodies. Filtration of toxins is absolutely critical for good health. That's why our bodies have been designed so that the major percentage of blood being filtered by the liver is coming from the portal vein, which carries blood directly from the intestines. This blood coming from the intestines typically contains high levels of endotoxins, exotoxins, microorganisms and allergens along with other nutrient substances.

When the liver is operating efficiently, it will clear 99% of toxins during the first pass. However, an overloaded or damaged liver will be inefficient at fully clearing these toxins, allowing them to re-circulate through the body causing inflammatory or toxic reactions.

2) **Secretory:**

The liver manufactures and stores bile in the gallbladder. Bile is a yellowy green fluid that contains amongst other chemicals bilirubin, a degradation product of haemoglobin. Bile is necessary for the emulsification of fats and facilitates the absorption of fat-soluble vitamins A, D, E and K, from the intestines. Bile is what gives faeces its yellow colour.

Bile also serves as a carrier for the elimination of modified toxins from the liver. In the intestines, the bile along with its toxic metabolites are absorbed by fibre from the diet and excreted as faeces. However, a diet low in fibre results in re-absorption of the bile acids and its toxins. This problem is further magnified when bacteria in the bowels digest these bile acids into even more damaging endotoxins.

***Your Liver:* The hardest working organ in your body**

Your liver is a vital organ that performs over 500 daily functions essential to health and wellbeing including:

- ✓ Filtering toxins, chemicals and metabolic by-products out of your body.
- ✓ Manufacturing thousands of new body proteins including enzymes, hormones, cellular organelles and numerous chemicals, essential to good health.
- ✓ Producing bile (a yellow liquid) to help in the digestion and absorption of fats and fat-soluble vitamins.
- ✓ A storage facility for vitamins and minerals and sugar as glycogen, for the production of quick energy when needed.

Due to the enormous number of vital functions carried out by the liver, it is essential to have it functioning at optimal capacity for vibrant health.

3) **Metabolic:**

The liver performs a multitude of metabolic functions including:

- Carbohydrate, protein and fat metabolism
- Storage of vitamins and minerals such as iron, copper, vitamins B12, A, D, E, and K.
- Conversion of beta-carotene into vitamin A.
- Activates vitamin D.
- Neutralises drugs, chemicals, hormones and other metabolic by-products for safe elimination.
- Aids immunity, as in destroying micro-organisms via its specialised kupffer cells.
- The manufacture of co-agulation factors needed for blood clotting.

Our liver takes the brunt of our lifestyle. Too much alcohol, smoking and a diet high in processed and fatty foods, along with environmental toxins and medications can put a real load on the liver. Everything that you breathe and eat that is broken down and absorbed into the bloodstream, or absorbed through the skin, passes through the liver. It is the liver's job

How might you know if you are suffering from a clogged, overworked liver?

If you have any of the following symptoms your liver is most likely to be in need of help with cleansing and detoxification:

- Fatigue
- Headaches
- Memory problems
- Digestive problems
- Allergies
- Aches and pains
- Acne or skin rashes
- Obesity
- Dark circles under your eyes
- Poor circulation especially in hands and feet
- Back pain
- Redness on palms
- Lack-lustre hair
- Insomnia
- Unusual body odour and bad breath
- High cholesterol
- Any diagnosed diseases
- Vertigo or dizziness
- Depression and mood swings
- Fluid retention.

If you can relate to any of these symptoms, your liver may be calling out for attention.

to render harmless any toxins and chemicals that could otherwise cause damage to body tissues.

If your liver becomes overwhelmed with this influx of toxins and chemicals, the overloaded liver will be inefficient at clearing them and so, they can continue to circulate throughout the body, causing disruption and damage before eventually being stored mainly in the fat cells of your organs and tissues. Depending on the type of toxin held in the body, you can experience all sorts of chronic or degenerative conditions that ultimately have their genesis in an overwhelming build-up of toxic accumulations that result from an overworked liver.

Cleansing your liver will essentially help it to detoxify your entire body, so it makes sense that in order to detoxify your body it is best to cleanse and support the organ that is actually responsible for body detoxification – your liver.

Over the years, I have successfully treated thousands of patients by always cleansing and supporting their livers as part of their treatment plan. Time and again I witnessed my clients transform their persistent ailments into real and lasting healing and with greatly improved energy levels, simply by cleansing and detoxifying their livers.

With a clean healthy functioning liver you can:

- Flush away unhealthy cholesterol
- Clear up your skin so it looks radiant again
- Shed excess weight
- Clear a fuzzy brain so your mind is alert once again
- Restore flexibility to your joints
- Improve your digestion
- Feel energised and alive
- And generally transform your health….

How does the liver detoxification system work?

The liver is an incredibly complex and efficient system that converts endotoxins (produced in the body), exotoxins (from outside the body) and other wastes into less damaging substances, which can then be eliminated from the body. In order for them to be eliminated, they must first be made water soluble, which makes it possible for the body to then eliminate them through the kidneys, the bowels and the sweat glands.

The liver accomplishes this task through a series of complex pathways know as **Phase 1** and **Phase 2** detoxification pathways.

The first stage of liver detoxification is called Phase 1 and it involves over 75 special enzymes that are known as the **Cytochrome P450 system**.

When Cytochrome P450 enzymes metabolize a toxin it chemically transforms it into either:

- A water soluble substance that can be easily excreted via the kidneys or as a component of bile. An example of a substance being treated by Phase 1 enzymes is caffeine, which can be made water soluble for direct excretion in the urine without having to go through the Phase 2 detoxification process.
- Converts it into a more chemically active metabolite ready for phase 2 detoxification. Some of these metabolites produced during the phase 1 detoxification process can be very toxic or even carcinogenic. For this reason, it's very important that the phase 2 detoxification system is up to task so that these dangerous metabolites can be safely neutralized before they cause any harm within the body.

As a consequence of the chemical reactions that take place during the phase 1 detoxification process, there is an increase in free radical production and so high levels of antioxidants (e.g. vitamins A, C, E and selenium) are needed to neutralize these damaging substances. In fact, both phase 1 and phase 2 detoxification systems involves many different enzymatic pathways, each dependent upon good nutrition to function properly.

After the toxins or chemicals have been processed by the phase 1 detoxification pathway, they are then subjected to a different set of enzymes called the "phase 2" detoxification pathway. Phase 2 attempts to convert these intermediate reactive metabolites from their fat-soluble state, into water-soluble substances so they can be easily excreted in the urine or as a component of bile. This conversion is achieved through a process known as 'conjugation', where various protein molecules and other substances are attached to these intermediate metabolites making them water soluble and therefore safe to be eliminated.

There are six different conjugation pathways in phase 2 detoxification. One of them: 'Glutathione conjugation' is considered the most important pathway, but this is not to say the other five pathways do not play an important role; they all need to be functioning optimally for good health.

Indeed, both phases in liver detoxification have to be properly supported with optimal amounts of key nutrients for detoxification to proceed smoothly. Vitamins and minerals are used in many of the enzymes involved in phase 1 and phase 2 detoxification, especially the B-vitamins. Antioxidants such as vitamins A, C and E are required to neutralize free radicals. Vitamin E and the mineral selenium are used as co-factors for glutathione peroxidase, a powerful antioxidant that protects against damage by free radicals and lipid peroxidation. Other nutrients vital to efficient detoxification in the phase 2 pathways includes the amino acids: cysteine, glycine, glutamine, methionine and taurine.

As I have previously emphasized throughout this book, only a high quality diet along with specific nutritional supplementation are needed to provide you with the necessary nutrients required for proper detoxification to take place. When nutrition is compromised through poor dietary and lifestyle choices, this will impede the liver's detoxification pathways, and invariably other organs will suffer as the body retains these toxins.

Unfortunately in today's world, most individual's Phase 1 and Phase 2 detoxification pathways are out of balance. This occurs due to micro-nutrient deficiencies and the problem is exacerbated when an individual is exposed to large amount of toxins or exposed to toxins over a long time period. As a result, the essential nutrients required for Phase 2 pathways to operate efficiently, get quickly depleted and so Phase 2 can no longer detoxify effectively to keep up with the incoming toxic metabolites from Phase 1.

This results in a build-up of highly reactive metabolites from Phase 1 pathways that can escape into the general circulation causing tissue damage and ultimately disease.

What makes things worse is the fact that such metabolites produced by Phase 1 detoxification are often-times, much more toxic than the original toxins being treated. This is why it is essential that both Phase 1 and Phase 2 detoxification pathways are always kept in balance, hence the need for good nutrition.

There is a term given to individuals whose Phase 1 and Phase 2 pathways are out of balance; such people are called "**Pathological Detoxifiers**". They can be identified as those individuals who are highly sensitive to smells, particularly paints, perfumes, cigarette smoke and most fumes. They can react adversely to pharmaceutical medicines and synthetic supplements. Their symptoms are often vague and ever-changing, ranging from constant fatigue, pains throughout the body, headaches and insomnia, to digestive ailments, anxiety and depression, skin rashes; none of which can be pinpointed to any single cause.

Great health benefits come from stimulating both Phase 1 and Phase 2 detoxification pathways, not only for Pathological Detoxifiers but also for everyone in general. With the right dietary choices, nutritional and herbal medicine support, individuals can finally get relief from their nagging ailments.

Due to every person's unique individual and biochemical makeup my suggestion is to consult a natural therapist who has an intimate knowledge in the underlying causes and treatment protocols for liver detoxification impairment. This will be your quickest and safest route to regaining health, especially if you feel you're a pathological detoxifier. I say this because of the many variables which combine to create this condition; there is no one-size-fits-all approach. Each person needs to be individually assessed to determine the best treatment strategy.

During the course of your treatment, these variables will usually change and so it is imperative to follow up with repeat appointments for the therapist to track this dynamic change and adjust treatments accordingly, for you to benefit fully and achieve a long lasting recovery.

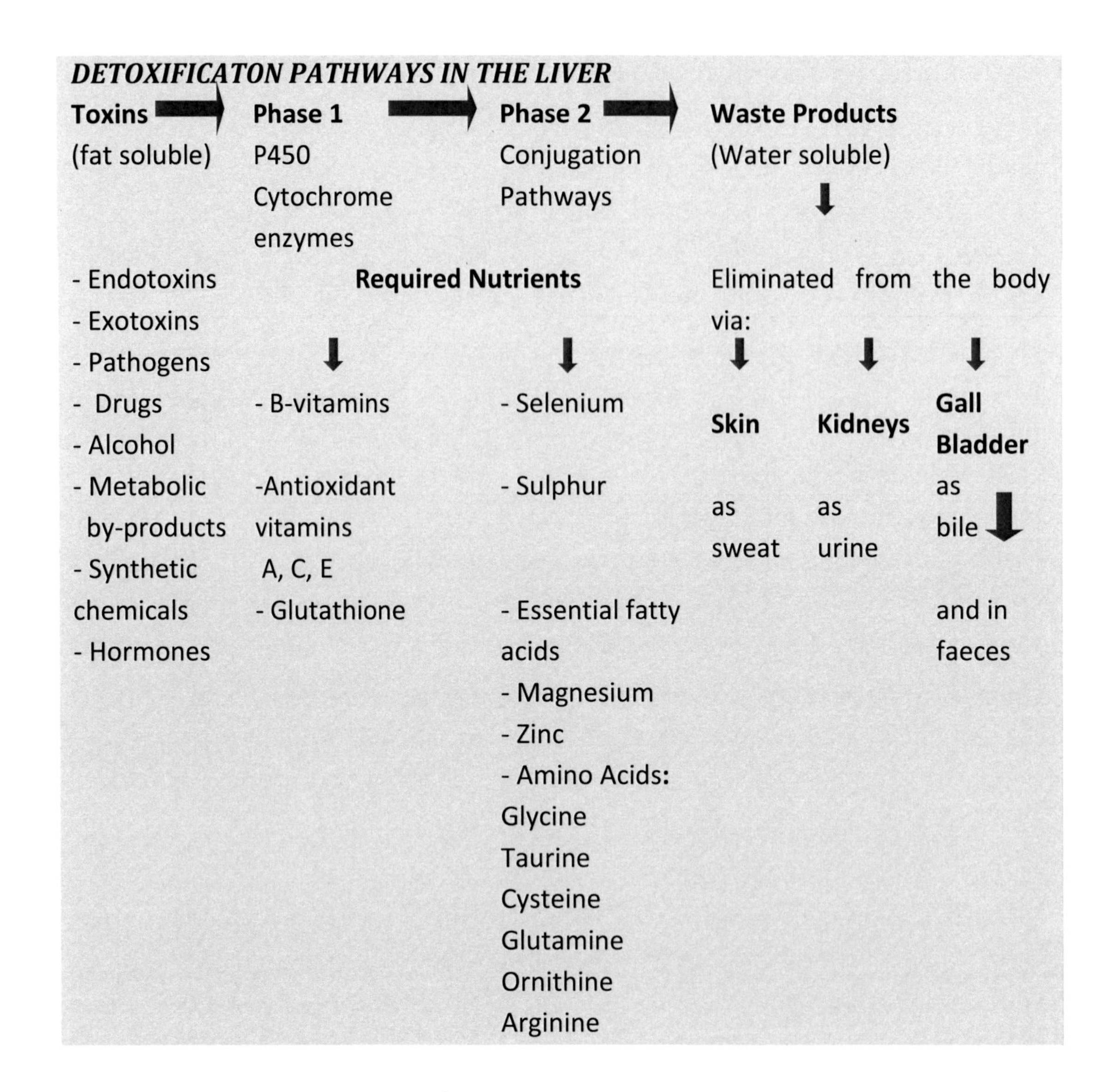

Tips for improving Liver Detoxification

There are many foods that nourish, protect and cleanse the liver while also supporting both Phase 1 and Phase 2 detoxification pathways. They include:

- The Brassica family, i.e. cabbage, broccoli and brussels sprouts. These vegetables contain many beneficial nutrients and chemical constituents that are used by the liver. One notable compound they contain in "Indole-3-Carbinol", a very active stimulant of Phase 2 liver enzymes and also a powerful anti-cancer agent.

- Other cruciferous vegetables of the Brassica family such as cauliflower, kale, radishes, turnips, watercress and bok choy contain many phytochemicals including glucosinolates, which are used by the liver to produce enzymes for Phase 1 and 2 detoxification.
- Asparagus contains amino acids that boost levels of two key Phase 2 enzymes that help break down alcohol. These amino acids remain stable even after high-temperature cooking, so asparagus remains a powerful allay even after steaming, boiling or roasting.
- Beetroot, globe artichoke, eggplant (aubergine), brown rice and spinach contain various phytonutrients including the B-vitamins which improve liver function and promote liver decongestion.
- Oranges and tangerines (but not grapefruits) contain limonene, a phytochemical that is a strong inducer of both Phase 1 and Phase 2 detoxification enzymes.

  Grapefruit on the other hand, contains naringenin, a substance which inhibits Phase 1 enzymes.

  Interestingly, people who are in the category of Pathological Detoxifiers may actually find it useful to include grapefruit juice in their diet. The rationale being, as previously mentioned, Phase 1 detoxification can turn harmless chemicals into very toxic or even carcinogenic metabolites. For this reason, it can be useful to slow down Phase 1 pathways to allow the Phase 2 detoxification to catch up.

  Caution is advised though if one is taking certain medications especially Warfarin, as to slow down Phase 1 activity will automatically increase the half-life of some drugs, causing them to remain active longer, thereby leading to possible life-threatening toxic side-effects.

- Eat some curry! The turmeric spice in curry powder contains a substance called curcumin that protects the liver from free radical damage, improves bile flow and stimulates Phase 2 pathways. Turmeric spice has anti-inflammatory properties and contributes to the production of glutathione, a potent liver-protective antioxidant used in Phase 1 & 2 detoxification pathways.

- Avocados are also a rich source of glutathione. Note, that dietary glutathione in foods appears to be efficiently absorbed into the blood. However, the same may not be true for glutathione supplements.
- Albion family vegetables for example, garlic, onions and shallots have sulphur-containing phytonutrients that activate Phase 2 detoxification pathways.

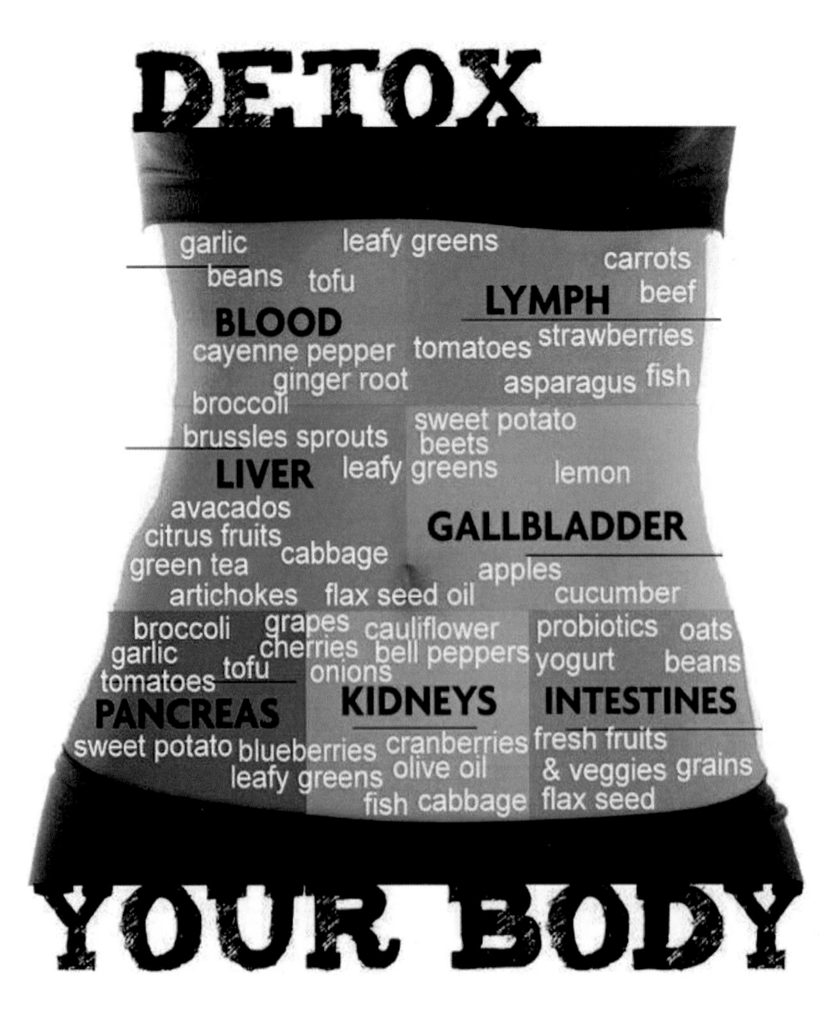

Nutritional Factors to Optimise Liver Function

- Lecithin granules are a complex mixture of chemical compounds called phospholipids that are obtained from soya beans. Lecithin helps to remove fat and cholesterol build-up in your liver, so it can do a better job detoxifying harmful chemicals and toxins from your body. Choline and inositol are the main phospholipids of Lecithin that are very effective for liver function and for the regulation of fat metabolism.
- B-complex vitamins are needed as co-factors in Phase 1 detoxification enzymes. The antioxidant vitamins A, C and E are also quite important in protecting the liver from free radical damage as well as helping in detoxification. The minerals calcium, magnesium, selenium, sulphur, zinc and potassium are also used by the detoxification enzymes as co-factors to facilitate the process of detoxification by the liver.

Botanical Medicines beneficial to the Liver

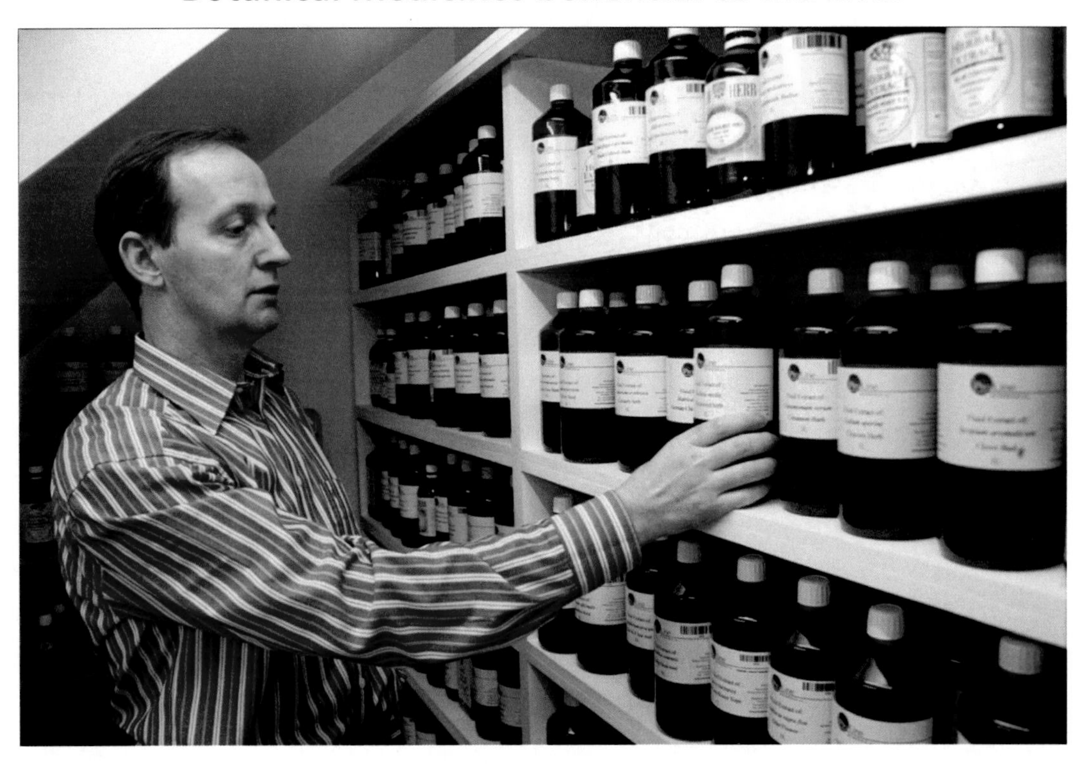

There are many herbs that contain various phytonutrients that have been shown to boost the activity of key detoxifying liver enzymes while also providing antioxidant protection against free radicals being produced during the detoxification process.

Some examples include:

- **St Mary's Thistle (Silybum marianum):** This herb is backed up with impressive research into one of its flavonoid compounds: 'silymarin'. Silymarin has been shown to protect hepatocytes (liver cells) from damage while also enhancing the detoxification process. It can do this by a number of mechanisms:
    - Acts as an antioxidant to neutralize free radicals produced during Phase 1 detoxification. Silymarin is many times more potent than the antioxidant vitamins A, C and E.
    - Increases the production of glutathione and also prevents its depletion. Glutathione is needed for Phase 2 detoxification enzymes.
    - Increases the rate of liver tissue regeneration by stimulating protein synthesis.

  St Mary's Thistle contains many other phytonutrients including bitter principles that stimulate bile secretion and improve digestion in general. Germany's Commission E, a governmental agency that reviews the safety and effectiveness of herbal medicines approved the use of St. Mary's Thistle as a treatment for toxic liver disease and a supportive treatment for chronic inflammatory liver disease and cirrhosis of the liver.(37)

- **Globe Artichoke (Cynara scolymus)**: This garden vegetable has similar liver protective and regenerating properties to St. Mary's Thistle. These properties are ascribed to the plant's constituent, cynarin. Globe Artichoke stimulates the flow of bile from the liver to the gallbladder where toxins can be removed. If bile stays around the liver tissues, a condition called jaundice occurs and this can cause liver damage. This plant has also been shown to keep cholesterol and triglyceride levels (blood fats) within the healthy range. It helps prevent the formation of gallstones and is used in conditions where there is liver cell damage, gallbladder disease and gallstones.

- **Turmeric (Curcuma longa):** This yellow culinary root has been the most clinically tested and written about herb for its anti-inflammatory properties. Since most chronic health problems are inflammatory in nature I often include this excellent liver remedy in my herbal tonics. Curcumin, the yellow pigment that gives turmeric its colour, exhibits a variety of biological activities on the liver, including protecting it from free radical damage while also stimulating bile flow. Research done on liver cancer showed that curcumin inhibits cancer cell growth and also triggers cancer cell death (apoptosis).

- **Dandelion Root (Taraxacum officinale):** This common garden herb is widely regarded by herbalists as the supreme liver cleanser. It stimulates liver functions and bile flow and has gently laxative properties. In animal research, dandelion was shown to increase both Phase 1 and Phase 2 detoxification enzymes in their livers. The whole plant is also a good source of most vitamins along with iron, zinc and potassium. It is traditionally used by herbalists to treat fatty livers, cirrhosis and toxic overload.

- **Burdock (Arctium lappa)**: The root of this plant is a favourite blood and liver cleanser among herbalists. It stimulates bile flow and helps purify the blood due to its diuretic effect. It also has mild laxative properties. These properties make Burdock especially useful in conditions where an accumulation of toxic metabolites are present in the body, in particular, skin diseases such as eczema, psoriasis, acne, boils, rashes, etc.

There are many other herbs shown to exhibit protective and restorative actions on damaged liver tissue; enhance both Phase 1 and Phase 2 pathways, improve bile flow and cleanse clogged up livers. Examples include: Andrographis, Astragalus, Barberry, Bupleurium, Dan shen, Greater celandine, Schizandra and Yellow dock.

All of these herbs also have additional properties including, immune-stimulating effects, digestive stimulants and laxatives, blood cleansing and diuretic effects, cardiovascular tonics and blood sugar normalisers. I prescribe different herbs based on individual requirements.

Whilst improving one's diet and including the aforementioned foods and supplements, is an absolute must to help a poor functioning liver, I would also recommend an individualised herbal tonic that includes some of the aforementioned liver herbs. Such a tonic not only supports and protects the liver but ensures that even the most sluggish of livers can function again at an optimal level. Not only will you get your liver functioning better as a result and with improved digestion, but you will also have increased energy levels and an overall sense of wellbeing.

CHAPTER 5

BLOOD CLEANSING

> *"Healing is an inside job" – Dr. B.J. Palmer*

In addition to having efficient bowel and liver detoxification for good health, blood cleansing is also very important for the overall health of your body.

Our blood is a viscous fluid that is thicker and more adhesive than water. It has a temperature of 38 degrees centigrade with a pH range of 7.35 – 7.45 (slightly alkaline). It is composed of 45% formed elements (i.e. red and white blood cells) and 55% plasma (watery liquid containing water, proteins and an array of other solutes.

Our blood is also filled with many impurities including metabolic end-wastes, environmental toxins including heavy metals (e.g. arsenic, lead, mercury, aluminium, etc.) as well as an over-abundance of circulating dietary fats and cholesterol. All these impurities must be continually removed from the blood stream to maintain optimal health.

Blood has three basic functions:

1. The transportation of oxygen, nutrients, hormones and enzymes to every cell in the body and also to carry away metabolic waste products, carbon dioxide, pathogens and any other toxins for excretion.
2. The regulation of:
    a. The pH via various buffer systems
    b. Body temperature

   c. The water content of body cells via dissolved sodium ions.
3. Protection against:
   a. Blood loss via clotting mechanisms
   b. Foreign microbes via circulating white blood cells

Blood Toxicity

Our liver and kidneys work continuously to cleanse the blood of impurities. Some additional cleansing of the blood is also carried out by the lungs via respiration, by the skin via sweating and by our colon via bile excretion in our stool.

Most sickness starts when toxins and metabolic wastes begin to accumulate in the blood. These impurities can disrupt the pH of the blood, which can lead to the weakening of the immune system.

When the immune system is in a weak state, the liver, kidneys and colon become impaired in their function. If these organs continue to operate at sub-optimal levels for any period of time, toxins that should otherwise be neutralized and eliminated may linger in the bloodstream resulting in the body becoming more susceptible to disease and ill health.

So, when embarking on a blood cleansing routine, it stands to reason that one should also support the liver, kidneys, colon, lungs and skin in their functions in order to help keep the blood clean. Many of the foods and herbs used to cleanse and improve liver detoxification are also excellent blood cleansers.

Herbal Blood Purifiers

There is a special class of herbs called **'Alteratives'** that are used to cleanse the blood and support the other organs of elimination. Alteratives are the classic detoxifying herbs, also commonly called "Blood Purifiers". They are used to bring about a gradual cleansing of the blood via their abilities to restore and maintain proper function to the organs of elimination. By their very nature, they work slowly and methodically so that over a period of some months, they cleanse the blood stream of accumulated wastes and toxins. There are many such herbs in the Alterative category but some notable examples include:

Burdock Root (Arctium lappa) I mentioned this herb in the liver detox section of this book, with its ability to stimulate bile flow thereby boosting the liver's capacity to remove toxins from the body via the bile. Burdock has proved to be an excellent alterative herb that cleanses the blood by increasing the effectiveness of all, the body's elimination systems. Its diuretic effect helps the kidneys filter impurities from the blood. Its gentle laxative effect helps purge the colon of its contents, preventing their re-absorption.

Due to its overall actions, Burdock Root has been a favourite amongst herbalists, having been traditionally used for centuries to clear the body of congestion and purify the blood.

Red Clover (Trifolium pratense) The blossoms of this herb have excellent blood purifying properties. They stimulate the liver to increase bile production and activate the gallbladder, which gives a laxative effect to the bowels. Red Clover also has a gently diuretic action on the kidneys helping to further cleanse the blood. It also works as an expectorant helping clear the lungs of accumulated phlegm and toxins.

Red Clover is also reputed to have anti-cancer properties, thus leading to its inclusion in some famous cancer-fighting herbal formulas such as Rene Caise's "Essiac" tonic, and the "Hoxsey" herbal formula.

Red Clover is also a good source of many essential nutrients including the B-vitamins, vitamin C, as well as several minerals (calcium, chromium, magnesium, potassium and phosphorus).

Stinging Nettles (Urtica dioica) If people only knew of all the health benefits that accrue, by regularly ingesting the common garden nettle, they might start growing them by the barrow load instead of treating them as a noxious weed and pouring weed killer over them.

As a young boy, I remember my mum recounting to us children, the time when she was a young girl, her parents raised turkeys to sell at the Christmas markets. A week or so before the turkeys where due to be sold, my mum's parents would feed nettle stew to the turkeys in order to make their gizzards a healthy bright red colour. Potential customers were immediately attracted to these healthy looking turkeys with the result that my grandparents always sold out of their stock within the first few hours each Christmas.

The entire nettle plant is of value, including the leaves, flowers, stem and roots. The health benefits attributed to nettles are legion but suffice to say, it is about the best blood purifier available. The ancient druids consumed nettles as part of their stable diet for thousands of years. They had them in stews, soups and as teas. They knew it to be a rich nutritive herb for making healthy blood. It's a circulatory stimulant and diuretic and also has anti-inflammatory properties. The plant can also lower blood sugar levels making it useful in diabetes. It also speeds up wound healing.

There are numerous other herbs that are useful blood cleansers, which I could elaborate upon, but it's outside the scope of this book. Herbs such as cleavers, poke root, sarsaparilla and yellow dock, to name only a few that are depuratives, laxatives, diuretics and lymph cleansers. Such herbs along with many others, can be employed in the treatment of many chronic health conditions by virtue of their depurative (blood purging) actions.

More Blood Cleansing Treatments:

Oral Chelation Therapy

Chelation (Greek work for "claw") therapy was developed during World War II as a technique for removing heavy metal toxins from the bodies of soldiers exposed to chemical warfare and also for the ship builders exposed to high levels of lead that were in the paints used to paint the ships at that time.

These days chelation therapy can be utilized to treat acute heavy metal poisoning as well as cardiovascular conditions such as atherosclerosis (hardening of the arteries) because it reduces the amount of plaque-causing calcium in the blood.(38)

Chelation therapy involves the removal of heavy metals from the bloodstream via the administration of certain binding agents (chelating agents) – most commonly the synthetic amino acid EDTA (ethylenediaminetetraacetic acid), which binds with metals and other toxins and excretes them in the urine. It is usually administered via an intravenous drip to individuals suffering from acute heavy metal poisoning.

Although chelation therapy as practiced today is a very effective way of cleansing the blood vessels of heavy metals and calcium deposits including excess cholesterol, it requires the services of specialist doctors to administer and generally costs an arm and a leg!

However, the good news is we don't need to do that. We can do a much cheaper safer non-surgical and non-medical form of chelation by oral means.

Studies have shown that the fresh leaves of the coriander plant can mop up and flush out heavy metals such as lead, mercury and aluminium from the body. According to Jon Barrow, a Naturopath and author of "Lessons from the Miracle Doctors", consuming 400mg of coriander a day can clean the body of heavy metals (particularly those located in the cardiovascular system) in as little as 2-3 weeks.(39) He recommends making up a coriander pesto and consuming two teaspoonfuls daily for a period of three weeks. If you do this a few times per year, you'll maintain clean flexible arteries.

Dr. David Williams shares a great recipe for a coriander pesto in his June '98 "Alternatives" newsletter. Here it is:

Coriander Pesto

- 1 clove of garlic
- ½ cup of either: almonds, cashews, hazelnuts or macadamia nuts (raw & soaked). (Alternatively, use nut butters from health stores).
- 1 cup of packed fresh coriander leaves (approx. 140g).
- 2 tablespoons of lemon juice (36ml).
- 6 tablespoons of organic olive oil (110ml).

Method:

Put the coriander and olive oil in a blender and chop it. Add the rest of the ingredients and blend to a lumpy paste. You can add a little hot water if it's too lumpy.

Eat two teaspoonfuls of the pesto daily for a period of about three weeks to flush out any heavy metals including any calcium deposits that end up in calcified blood vessels (a primary cause of high blood pressure). I recommend you repeat this process three times a year as a good blood cleansing strategy and to achieve and maintain lovely clean and flexible blood vessels and so therefore, never have a need for blood pressure medication.

*** A word of caution** though for those of you whose bodies may be loaded with a lot of heavy metals. When you start ingesting the coriander pesto, the coriander may mobilize more heavy metals that it can safely carry out of your body. These heavy metals can potentially cross the blood-brain barrier, causing neurological damage.

To avoid this re-intoxification scenario, I recommend you also take ½ teaspoonful (2,000mg) of chlorella powder mixed in a little water 30 minutes before taking the coriander pesto.

Chlorella is a single-celled green micro-algae that gets its name from its high chlorophyll content (more than twice that of spirulina). Chlorella is extremely cleansing and is known for its ability to soak up, and expel heavy metals and pesticides from the body. So, chlorella is great for mopping up any excess heavy metals left floating around the bloodstream as a result of taking the coriander pesto.

Another excellent chelator is malic acid. This acid is found in apples and apple cider vinegar. Malic acid is particularly good at removing aluminium from the body. Aluminium tends to be high in people suffering from fibromyalgia and Alzheimer's. So the old saying:*"an apple a day keeps the doctor away"* certainly holds some truth. Also, the pectin in apples binds to cholesterol and so is useful in keeping high cholesterol at bay.

If you think your body is not loaded with many toxic metals, then consider the following:

- Do you have a mouthful of silver-amalgam fillings (mercury)?
- Did you get many vaccinations including the seasonal flu shot (mercury, aluminium)?
- Do you live in a polluted environment (lead, cadmium, etc.)?
- Do you smoke (cadmium, arsenic and over 4,000 polycyclic hydrocarbons)?
- Do you drink fluoride water?
- Do you regularly eat non-organic food (high in pesticides, herbicides, etc.)?

The sad fact is we are all suffering from toxic overload. There is nowhere we can go in the world today that is free from pollution and other environmental challenges. All this exposure to pollution and heavy metals along with unhealthy lifestyle choices makes us humans the most toxic species on this planet!

Oil Pulling

Another excellent method of cleansing the bloodstream of toxins is by doing an ancient Ayurvedic therapy called "Oil Pulling" The process involves swishing a tablespoonful of vegetable oil around the mouth for a period of 20 minutes each morning, on an empty stomach and then spitting it out. The premise is that this action "pulls" out bacteria and their mycotoxins as well as other pathogenic micro-organisms and toxic debris.

As simple as it sounds, oil puling has been shown to have a very powerful cleansing and detoxifying effect, not only for oral health but also as a blood cleanser and systemic body detoxifier. If I were to use an analogy, I would compare the process of oil pulling to working the same way as soap. Soap is basically a type of fat that has a detergent effect. It attracts and dissolves non-polar (without electrical charge) molecules such as oil and grease. Likewise oil pulling attracts other non-polar molecules such as the fatty membrane of bacteria and other germs located in the mouth.

So, as the oil gets swished around the teeth and gums, any bacteria hiding along the gum line and between the teeth gets flushed out and dissolved into the oil. In addition, when the oil is repeatedly swished around the mouth, the salivary glands are stimulated to secrete saliva. This salivary fluid contains, in addition to enzymes, many toxins and chemicals, which are absorbed directly from the blood, due to the nature of the capillaries surrounding the salivary glands, being quite porous and allowing these toxins to enter.

After 20 minutes of swishing, sucking and pulling the oil through the teeth and around the mouth, this heterogeneous mixture of oil, saliva, toxins and disease-causing micro-organisms turns into a slimy white liquid, which is then discarded by spitting it out and immediately afterwards washing the mouth out with salty water.

Ukrainian physician, Dr. F. Karach, who reintroduced Oil Pulling Therapy to the western world back in 1992, claimed that it can alleviate numerous health problems ranging from digestive disorders and skin conditions to hormonal problems and even heart disease. He said it cured his arthritis within three days and also cured him of a chronic blood disorder he suffered for fifteen years.(40)

He postulates that oil pulling works by cleansing and detoxifying the body of disease-causing pathogens and their mycotoxins, and as a consequence health problems of all types can be cured. In his clinical practice he teaches 'oil pulling' to his patients with great success.

I must say that it's one of the most remarkable methods of detoxification that I've come across in my career as a Naturopathic physician. I've now been doing oil pulling therapy for the past year and I first noticed an improvement in my dental health. My teeth became whiter and my gums are now a healthy pink and no longer bleed when flossing. Also, my skin has become smoother with a clearer complexion. That alone makes it worthwhile.

SOME POSITIVE EFFECTS OF OIL PULLING INCLUDE:

- Plaque prevention
- Prevention of tooth cavities
- Prevention of gingivitis (bleeding of gums)
- Prevention of halitosis (bad breath)
- Aids in overall detoxification
- Reduces inflammation
- Clears up sinus congestion
- Relief from skin conditions (acne, eczema, rashes)
- Supports normal liver and kidney function
- Pain reduction

Oil Pulling Method

Step 1

In the morning, before breakfast and before drinking any liquids including water, you take one tablespoonful of vegetable oil in your mouth making sure not to swallow it. The recommended oils to use are Sunflower or Sesame oil. Dr Bruce Fife N. D. in his book "Oil Pulling Therapy" recommends Coconut oil to be the best choice due to its anti-microbial properties, however it's more expensive. Other proponents of oil pulling claim that any vegetable oil will work.

Step 2

Move the oil around your mouth in a swishing motion, sucking and pushing it through your teeth for a period of 20 minutes, taking care not to swallow any oil. Swishing activates the salivary glands thereby drawing more toxins out of the blood. As the oil becomes saturated with micro-organisms and toxic debris, it turns white in colour.

If, during the process, the oil causes you to gag or becomes too unpleasant, just spit it out and start again. Take another tablespoonful of oil and continue until you've pulled for a total of 20 minutes. After a few times doing it, you will find it easier to do, just like brushing your teeth really.

Step 3:

When 20 minutes of oil pulling have elapsed, spit the oil out and then rinse your mouth with warm salty water. The salty water is an effective anti-microbial and can sooth any mouth irritations. Finally, brush your teeth to dislodge any hidden bacteria or toxins that may still be left in your mouth.

Unlike other methods of detoxification that are typically done over short periods, oil pulling should become a regular part of your daily schedule. The process works best if done in the morning and it can be done every day or several times a week. What's more, it is cheap to do and is also a very safe form of detoxification.

CHAPTER 6

THE KIDNEYS, SKIN, LUNGS AND LYMPHATICS ROLE IN DETOXIFICATION

> *"We are much better off taking a daily approach and being supportive, to the cleansing organs that are designed to detoxify our bodies."*
>
> *– Dr. David K. Hill*

No body detoxification process would be complete without also addressing these four organ systems of drainage and elimination. When we embark upon a bowel and liver detoxification programme, we also need to make sure that we support all organs involved in drainage and elimination, otherwise we may experience symptoms of toxic backup. With this in mind, full and proper detoxification also includes the organs involved in drainage and elimination which are the kidneys, skin, lungs and the lymphatic system.

THE KIDNEYS

When the body's metabolic wastes along with other toxins are converted to water soluble compounds by the liver, they can then be safely eliminated from the body, primarily via the kidneys and also by the sweat glands of the skin. The more toxins we are exposed to, the greater the burden on our kidneys and over time the ability of the kidneys to excrete toxins diminishes. Also, when the kidneys do not have enough water, they cannot function properly. As a result tiny solid deposits can start to accumulate in the kidneys, leading to the formation of kidney stones.

There is a well-known saying in environmental law ***"the solution to pollution is***

dilution". While it's not exactly a panacea to solving all of the earth's pollution problems, this law can have its uses when applied with our health and kidneys in mind.

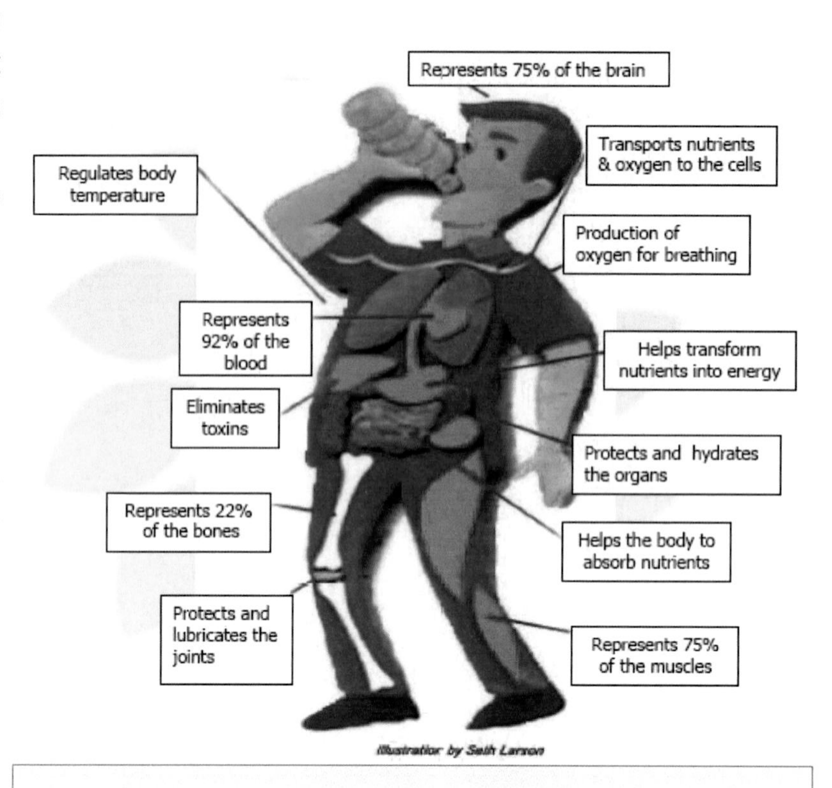

Illustration by Seth Larson

We need to flush toxins and the body's metabolic end-wastes away from the kidneys and the best way to do this is with plenty of clean filtered water. Like our planet, our bodies are about 70% water and every cell needs water to function in a healthy way. Water also hydrates our cells and helps flush away metabolic wastes being produced every second by our cells.

> ***As we grow old we lose the instinct to drink and gain the instinct to over eat. We must teach our bodies to drink more water and to eat less food, to eat more vegetables and less meat, and celebrate the meal.***

I'm often asked by my clients how much water does one need to drink? Well, when you take into consideration that each day you lose approximately two litres (8 glasses) of water through the kidneys, skin, lungs and bowel and that if this water is not replaced, you will become dehydrated. But that doesn't mean that you need to drink two litres of water daily.

For one thing, you can easily get one litre of water just from the food you eat, especially if you eat lots of fruits and vegetables. With this in mind, a healthy recommendation for water consumption would be around six glasses each day.

Of course, if you are involved in heavy strenuous exercise or live in a hot arid climate, you'll definitely need extra water to stay adequately hydrated. Also if you have any illness that includes fever, diarrhoea, or vomiting, you will need extra fluids too. As a general rule of thumb, if you are urinating several times a day and your urine is pale in colour, you should be okay.

Just as important as quantity is, as a prerequisite to proper detoxification, so also is quality when it comes to water intake. Purified water that is free from contaminants can better dissolve and remove toxins more easily from the body. Water in plastic bottles is best avoided as it often contains toxins that have leaked into the water from the plastic packaging. Investing in a high quality water filtration system such as a "Reverse Osmosis" water purifier that removes 98% of all chemical contaminants would be money well spent.

Drinking filtered water is possibly the best health enhancement habit you can develop and it is so simple; a glass of water every two hours. Alternatively, drinking herbal teas are also a wonderful way to hydrate the body and cleanse the kidneys. One example is dandelion tea as previously described in the liver detoxification section. Dandelion is a natural diuretic that works to cleanse and detox both the liver and kidneys. Other herbs that aid the kidneys include: cleavers, couch grass, celery, nettles, parsley and uva-ursi. Although caffeinated beverages such as tea, coffee and cola, along with alcohol act as diuretics, they also add to the body's toxin load and are best avoided and especially during a body cleanse.

THE SKIN

Did you know that your skin is the largest organ in the body and is capable of eliminating up to one kilogram of waste through its sweat pores each day? Research studies show that sweating can eliminate toxic substances including heavy metals from the body, thereby taking some of the pressure off the kidneys.(41) In fact natural health practitioners often refer to the skin as *"the third kidney"* and rightly so. The multitude of tiny sweat glands acts like small kidneys, removing toxins and cleansing the blood of health-destroying poisons.

If the pores in your skin become clogged up and can't function properly, this will place extra strain on the kidneys due to the extra load of toxins. An excellent way to rectify this problem is by a technique known as "Dry Skin Brushing".

Dry Skin Brushing

One of the best techniques for clearing out blocked skin pores and for encouraging lymphatic drainage is to do regular Dry Skin Brushing. Skin that gets clogged up with toxins and dead skin cells cannot function properly in eliminating such toxins.

Dry skin brushing on a daily basis is an extraordinary gentle yet powerful technique that will:

- Remove dead skin cells and unblock clogged pores allowing the skin to breath easily.
- Increase blood flow to the skin thereby helping your body to discharge toxic wastes.
- Increases blood flow to the skin, allowing more nourishment and oxygen to reach the skin.
- Stimulate the peripheral lymphatics to drain away metabolic wastes and toxins that have collected in the interstitial spaces between body cells.

Daily skin brushing will quickly relieve puffiness and give your skin a smooth feel with a radiant look. It consists of spending approximately three minutes each morning just before you shower or bath, brushing your skin all over, using a natural fibre, long-handled brush. The technique is simple: you start at your feet and brush up your legs using long sweeping strokes. Next, brush your hands and up your arms. Then brush across your upper back and up the back of your torso. Brush your abdomen, neck and upper chest in the direction of your heart. The reason I'm giving you these specific directions to brush, is so that you brush in the direction of lymph flow only.

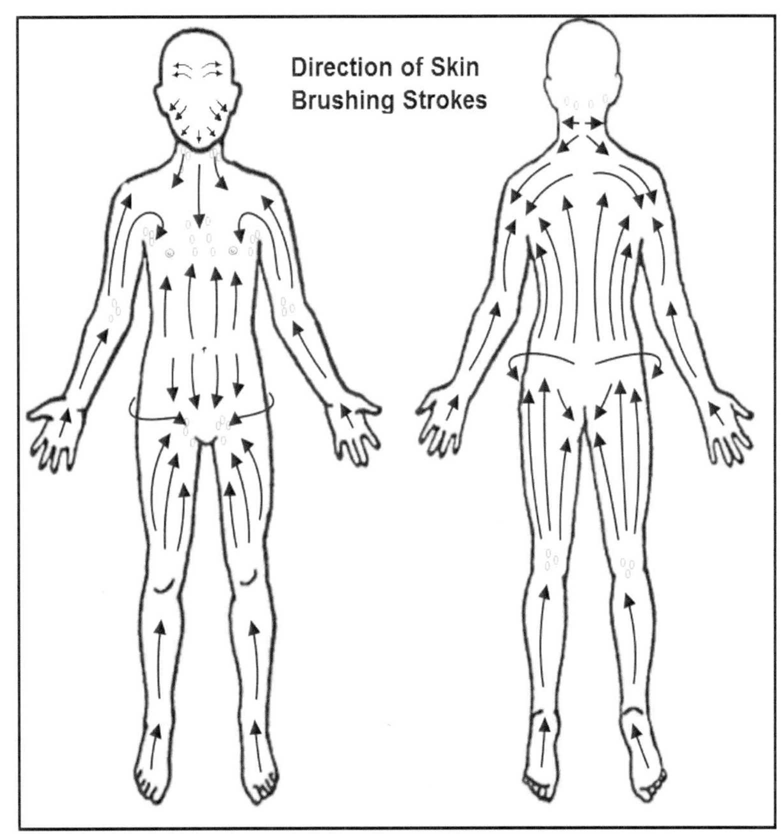

Do not brush your face as the brush is too rough for the delicate skin on your face, and also go gently on any other sensitive areas. Ideally, you should brush until your skin gets a warm glowing look, but do not brush so hard that your skin turns red or gets scratched. After dry skin brushing, take a shower or bath to wash away any dead skin cells. I also recommend that you clean the brush in warm soapy water every two weeks and also, don't share brushes for hygiene reasons.

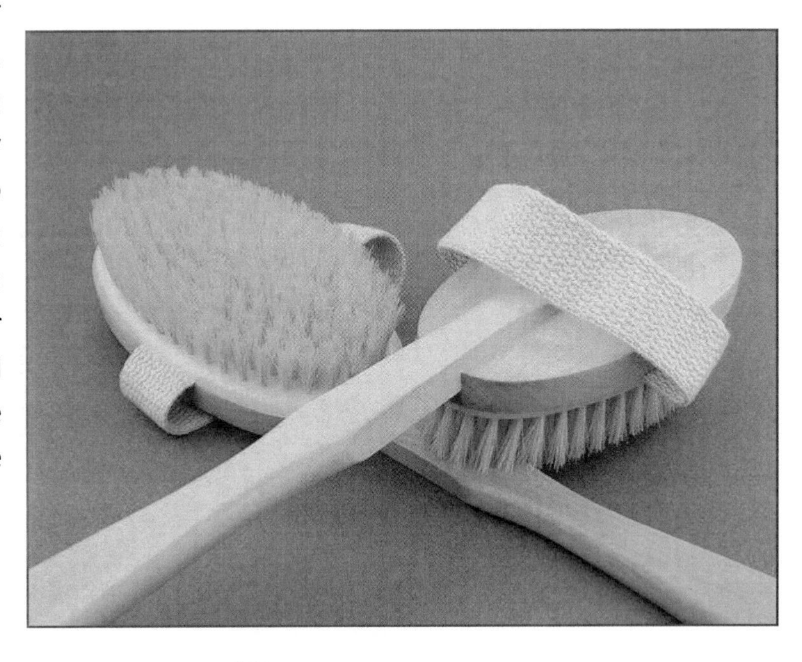

Sweat it Out

We've long known that sweating is not just a way to cool the body; it also has a very cleansing and detoxifying effect too. Research studies have shown that toxic substances including pesticides, heavy metals and many other fat-stored toxins are eliminated from the body through sweat. So it stands to reason that we should encourage our bodies to sweat more and thereby reap the health benefits of this simple bodily process.

Unfortunately, in our modern day culture sweating is perceived as an undesirable bodily function to be suppressed by every means. So we spray our bodies with antiperspirants loaded full of toxic aluminium, we live in air-conditioned buildings and mostly work in sedentary jobs.

Far-Infrared Sauna

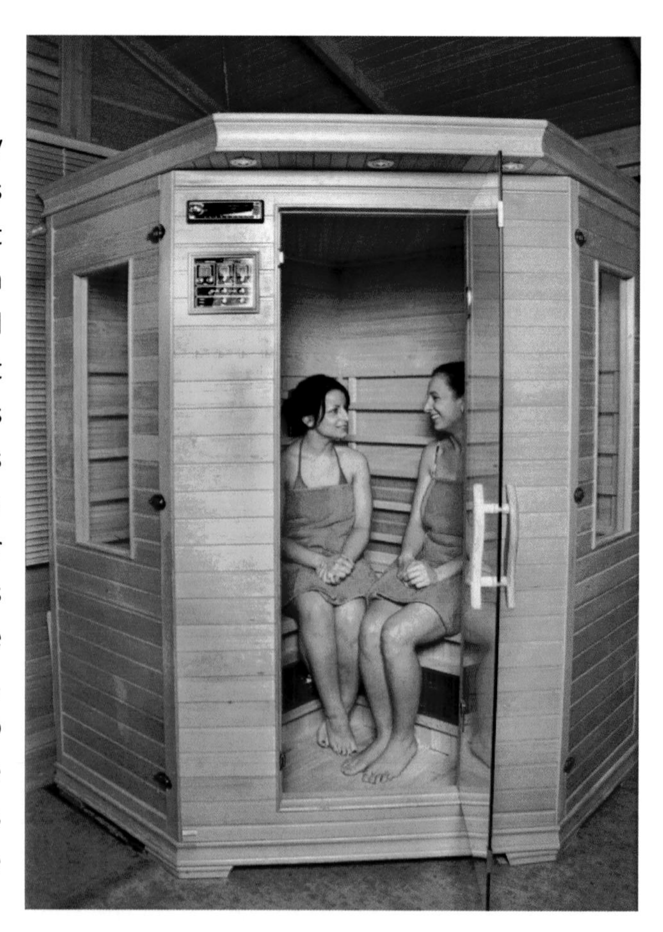

One way to induce sweating is by using a sauna. Research shows that Far-infrared saunas are most effective at inducing a detoxifying sweat. As opposed to traditional steam saunas that operate in excess of 75 degrees centigrade, far-infrared saunas generate radiant energy via electromagnetic waves at a lower temperature of 60-65^{0}C. This makes for a more comfortable sauna experience. In addition, radiant energy is able to penetrate more deeply into the skin and underlying fat cells causing the body to sweat more profusely.

Because of the deep penetration of far-infrared rays, these types of sauna produce a sweat composed of around 20% of toxins as compared to the sweat derived from using traditional steam saunas, which is composed of only 3% of toxins.(42) This superior detoxification through far-infrared therapy will go a long way to help relieve symptoms, boost your overall health and vitality and reduce or prevent future illness from ever arising. My recommendations are to have an infrared sauna once a week for an hour, as part of a health maintenance programme. If you are dealing with more significant health concerns, then twice or three times per week may be needed for a period.

The infrared sauna featured on the previous page is the one I have installed at my health centre and I find the ideal way to completely relax after a busy day at the office is to take some time to enjoy the intense warmth of its infra red rays. After just thirty minutes my blood circulation is stimulated and my body feels refreshed and revitalised, and some extra calories have been lost.

THE LUNGS

Like the other organs of elimination, the lungs too are also responsible for eliminating metabolic wastes including carbon dioxide and water. They act as a defence barrier to the billions of micro-organisms – bacteria, viruses and fungi – in the air you breathe. In addition, the lungs can alter the pH of the blood by controlling the saturation levels of carbon dioxide dissolved therein.

Of course, the primary function of the lungs is to supply all body cells with life-giving oxygen. It does this via the action of the diaphragm (a large sheet of strong muscle separating the chest and the abdominal cavity). When the diaphragm contracts, it moves downwards, toward the abdominal area, causing the chest to expand and suck in air. When the diaphragm relaxes, space in the chest cavity is reduced thus forcing air out of the lungs. This breathing process is controlled by the autonomic nervous system (without conscious control); however, it can be enhanced by conscious deep breathing.

Deep Breathing

Deep breathing for a few minutes several times a day has a tremendous effect at oxygenating the cells as well as boosting the circulation and improving lymph flow. Deep breathing forces the diaphragm downwards, creating negative pressure in the thorax (chest cavity) as well as increased intra-abdominal pressure, which together has the effect of powerfully promoting movement of blood within the large arteries and veins in these cavities. This in turn stimulates the whole circulation as well as encouraging circulation of lymph fluids, which transports toxic wastes away from the cells. Keeping your blood and lymph fluid moving efficiently is essential for good health. Deep breathing also has a calming and relaxing effect on the nervous system thus reducing the deleterious effects of stress on the body. Your blood pressure lowers. As your muscles let go of tension, your blood vessels dilate and your blood pressure can return to a normal level. Deep breathing triggers the release of endorphins, the body's feel-good chemicals, which improves feelings of well-being and provides pain-relief.

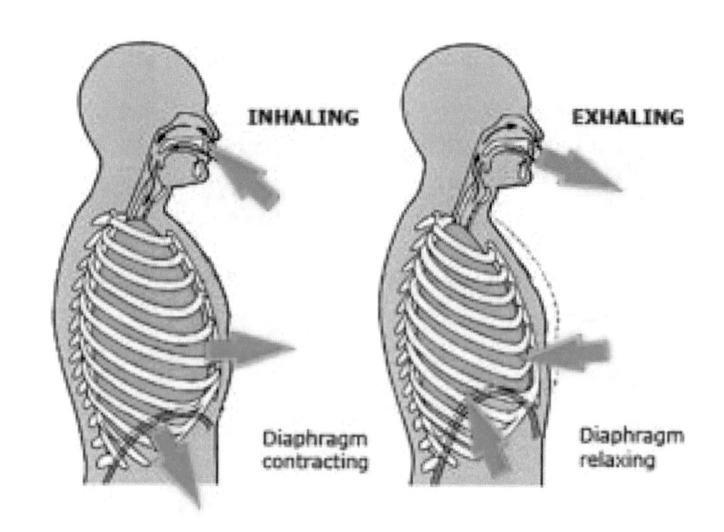

The process of deep breathing involves slow and deep inhalation through the nose while counting to six or eight, followed by a slow and complete exhalation for a similar count. When done properly, the abdomen should swell outwards while breathing in. Most people however, tend to breath shallow and therefore never fill the bottom part of their lungs. Deep breathing should be repeated for approximately ten breaths and performed several times a day to gain maximum benefit.

THE LYMPHATICS

Tiny blood vessels called capillaries constantly leak blood plasma (a clear liquid) into the tissue spaces between the cells of the body. In a sense the cells of our body float in a vast internal sea of liquid. This natural body fluid is called lymph. It is the job of the lymphatic system (a complex network of vessels and nodes), to drain away this lymph fluid from body tissues. Present in this lymph fluid are an array of metabolic wastes produced by cellular respiration, unwanted proteins, pathogens, and other toxins, which could not otherwise be removed from the body by other means. It is the job of the lymph nodes to inactivate and filter these micro-organisms and foreign substances that penetrate the body, which is why they have earned themselves the title, *"the garbage collectors"* of the body. After the lymph fluid has filtered through a series of lymph nodes, it eventually drains back into the bloodstream where it is excreted from the body via the urinary system.

Unlike the circulatory system that has the heart to pump the blood around, the lymphatic system doesn't have its own pump, so the movement of lymph fluid is dependent upon muscle contraction, diaphragmatic breathing and body movement. As muscles tighten, lymph vessels are squeezed and lymph fluid is pushed along and filtered through the lymph nodes on its way back to the venous blood supply. As a result, it is not uncommon to develop a sluggish lymphatic flow through inactivity, not drinking enough water and consuming the wrong types of food. The consequences of a poorly functioning lymphatic system will be a build-up of toxic wastes within the body tissues that ultimately lead to ill health and the development of chronic degenerative conditions.

WAYS TO TREAT LYMPHATIC CONGESTION

Exercise:

Since lymphatic flow is dependent on muscle contraction, one can see why regular exercise is necessary to ensure the lymph system flows properly. The human body is designed to be active and starts to malfunction if activity drops below a certain level. Joints stiffen up, muscles become weak and flabby and even the bones start to lose calcium and become brittle.

Regular exercise is the penultimate weapon in the quest to remain strong and healthy – it improves the capacity of the heart, circulation, lungs and lymphatic flow. One type of exercise that is especially good for the lymphatics is called rebounding.

Rebounding:

Rebounding is basically jumping on a mini-trampoline. A typical rebounder is three or four feet in diameter and about nine inches high. The vertical motion created by rebounding is more beneficial to lymphatic flow than horizontal motion such as running. The reason is that gravitational force is constantly changing while rebounding.

This change of force has a positive effect on the millions of one-way valves that allow lymph fluid to flow against gravity. The rhythmic bouncing on a rebounder causes all of the one-way valves to open and close simultaneously increasing lymph flow by as much as fifteen times. When rebounding on your mini-trampoline the aim isn't to bounce high, but to perform a series of small controlled jumps. In fact you will still get good results if you gently bounce up and down without your feet leaving the rebounder. The good thing about this type of exercise is that it is easy on your joints, very enjoyable and can be performed in your living room or the office.

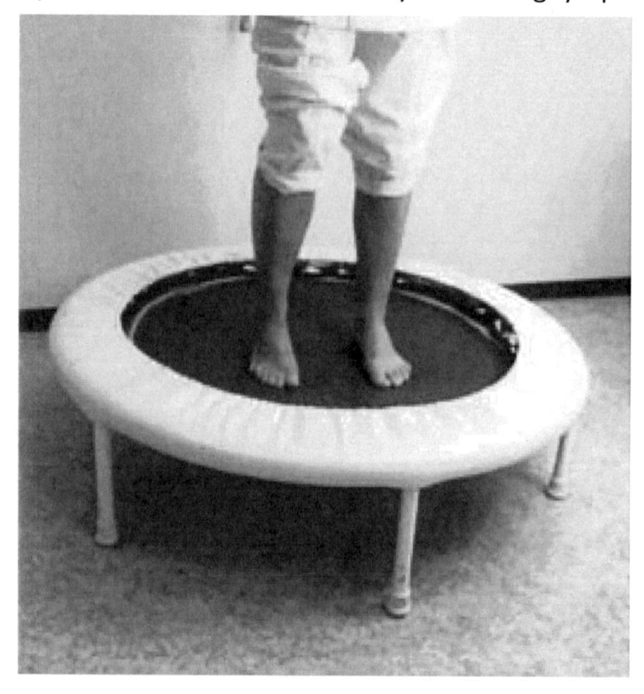

Lymphatic Drainage Massage:

This is a very gentle massage technique that is designed to stimulate the lymph's circulatory network in order to relieve blockages, speed up the removal of wastes and reduce water retention in the tissues. The technique involves the use of gentle rhythmic strokes and pumping movements where the skin is methodically stretched in the direction of the lymphatic flow to clear blockages, manually pump the lymph fluid and stimulate the lymph nodes.

I see a lot of clients at my clinic who suffer from a

LYMPH FACTS

- The body contains three times more lymph than blood. This lymphatic fluid is very important for protein metabolism and the immune system.
- The lymphatic system also helps to balance the electrical nature of the body and to stabilize the electrical transfer of energy.
- The lymph cycles through the body on a daily basis taking about 24 to 30 hours. This cycling through the body is accomplished by muscle contractions, which gently circulates the lymphatics through the body.
- The lymphatics then drain excess toxins and unneeded proteins, which are put back into the venous circulation and circulated through the liver and kidneys for disposal.
- When the lymphatics are sluggish, clogged, tight or tense, disease can ensue. Most of these diseases will include lymphatic swelling, itching of the skin, discolouration or blotching of the skin, general inflammation in the body, as well as fatigue and lethargy.
- It is very important that we cleanse the lymph through activity and exercise, and by minimizing toxic food, too much animal protein, fried foods and artery clogging fats.
- Lymphatic massage can also be very helpful in circulating the lymph.
- Infrared saunas and rebounders are also beneficial.

congested lymphatic system, so I usually do a few sessions of lymphatic drainage massage on them, and especially those suffering from fluid retention and the more chronic type of swelling known as 'lymphoedema' where limbs can swell up to twice or three times their normal size.

I've also applied lymphatic drainage massage with great success to conditions such as sports injuries, sinusitis, hormone imbalances in women, arthritis, fibromyalgia, chronic fatigue syndrome, fluid retention during pregnancy, in addition to also using it as a beauty treatment for the face and for reducing cellulite.

A Self-Care System of Lymph Draining

- Drain the head by tapping hard with the heels of both hands.
- Massage the indentations on the head behind the tops of the ears.
- Massage the centre of the forehead above the nose and drain off.
- Drain above and below the eyes in an outward direction into the side of the neck.
- Massage the points at the corners of the nose and mouth in a circular action and drain into the side of the neck.
- Pinch the jaws firmly up to the hairline.
- Drain from behind the top of the ears in a straight line down the side of the neck. Do this by drawing the fingers slowly but firmly along the skin to the collarbone.
- Place hands around the neck so that the tips of the fingers are almost touching the spine at the rear of the neck and the heels of the palm are almost touching at the front of the neck. Squeeze the back of the neck very rapidly five times. Without moving the hands, squeeze the front of the neck five times very rapidly.
- Drain the rear of the neck by tapping firmly.
- Dig the fingers into the arm pits while performing circular motions.
- Drain the front of the body by thumping the breast bone from shoulder to shoulder.

- Thump the heart area.
- Massage the liver vigorously with the heel of the hand. It is located on the right hand side of the stomach.
- Do the same with the pancreas, which is located on the left hand side of the stomach.
- Place the right hand under the right side at the base of the rib cage. Press firmly with the heel of the hand and bring firmly down to the navel. Repeat this five times.
- Place the heels of the hands on each side of the rib cage and with pressure, move both hands downward to meet the navel.
- Drain the back of the neck by rubbing downwards using the fingers of both hands.
- Drain shoulders (at rear) by thumping.
- Drain the lungs from the rear by thumping. (In the upper back).
- Drain the kidneys from the rear by thumping. (In the lower back).
- Work the fingers vigorously into both sides of the groin.
- Put both hands around the left ankle. With one thumb above the other, apply pressure (only with the thumbs) drawing the thumbs up the back of the leg to the groin.
- Now with the thumbs switched round to the front of the left ankle, repeat the process again.
- Drain the right leg as you did the left.
- With the flats of the fingers pressed gently into the back of both knees (at the popliteal nodes), squeeze firmly ten times.
- Stand on your tippy toes ten times.
- Take a deep breath and hold; force out the stomach, count to five and breathe out.
- When resting put up the feet to drain.

CHAPTER 7

ADDITIONAL CLINICAL DETOXIFICATION THERAPIES

"The part can never be well unless the whole is well" - Plato

Hopefully by now, you fully understand and appreciate the absolute necessity of having fully functioning detoxification and elimination systems as a prerequisite to achieving optimal health.

As we age these systems need ever more support via good nutrition, along with the therapies and practices I've already outlined. The good news though is to realise that you are not a helpless victim to the ravages of ageing and disease, but that you can in fact exercise considerable control over your own health and destiny. You can do this by using all available treatment methods at your disposal to strengthen and support your body in its detoxification role, and so prevent many diseases from occurring in the first place.

The following three therapies, i.e. Mud Wraps, Floatation and Light Therapy are additional treatments that I offer at my health centre, primarily due to their excellent detoxifying benefits and abilities to combat the effects of inflammation. As an added bonus, these treatments are most pleasurable for the client receiving them.

Mud Wraps

Mud wraps are the penultimate way to detoxify your body while also getting pampered simultaneously. Not only is it a luxurious and relaxing spa treatment to receive, this type of wrap also possesses impressive detoxifying properties with benefits including:

- Deep cleansing of the skin and its pores, leaving it smooth and glowing.
- Increases blood circulation throughout the body allowing for increased removal of toxins from tissues.
- Stimulation of the lymphatic system.
- The mud contains nutrients including trace minerals and vitamins, which are nourishing and rejuvenating to skin collagen.

The Treatment Process:

Although mud wrap treatments may vary from spa to spa, I offer a particular type of detox-wrap using a marine-based mud from the Yon-Ka range. This mud is noted for its deep cleansing and detoxifying qualities. It stimulates circulation, which aids in the removal of impurities and toxins for the body. It also replenishes the skin with essential minerals to leave the skin feeling soft and nourished.

Before the treatment begins, I prepare the massage table by covering it with a

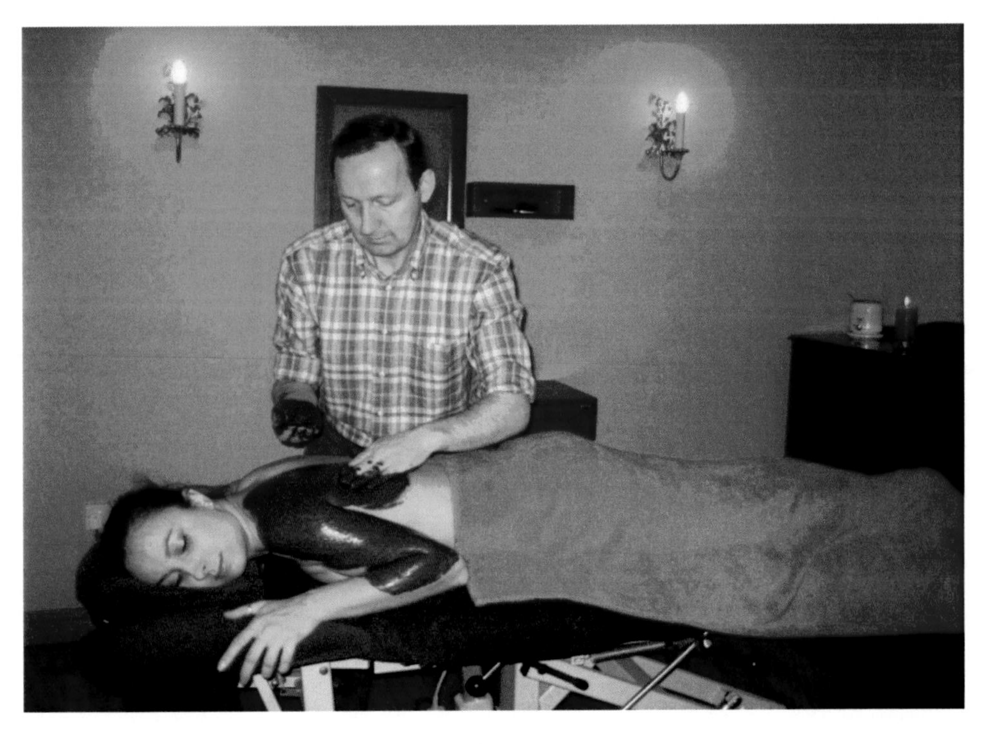

warm thermal blanket. On top of the blanket I then lay a sheet of aluminium foil and on top of that a sheet of plastic is laid out.

I start the mud wrap by first giving your body a thorough skin exfoliation (scrub) using a blend of sea salts mixed with a small volume of massage oil. All your dead skin cells will be removed, leaving your skin feeling velvety smooth. You then take a shower to rinse off the sea salts before the marine mud is applied.

Your whole body is then enveloped in warm marine mud and you are immediately wrapped up in the three layers of plastic sheeting, aluminium foil and finally the warm thermal blanket for maximum comfort and detoxifying effect.

The blanket's heat will induce sweating and you will remain covered for a period of thirty minutes for full effect. While wrapped, you will also be treated to a lymphatic facial and scalp massage.

After thirty minutes of intense sweating, the final step is to unwrap the sheeting and have a shower. Not only will you get an amazing detox treatment, your skin will also feel really smooth afterwards.

Floatation Therapy

At first glance floating may seem to be an odd sort of therapy, unlikely to yield many health benefits, or so I thought when I first came across it while living in Australia in the 1990's. I thought it would be too claustrophobic to be relaxing – one of its principle aims. Interestingly though, after about five minutes into my first float session, I found myself totally at ease in my watery environment. For the rest of my allotted hour my consciousness remained curiously suspended halfway between the waking and sleeping state, or as what scientists would call the 'hypnogogic' state. I was hooked on floating forever more….

Ever since having my first float all those years ago, whenever I now float, I quickly re-enter a realm of the deepest relaxation and bliss known only to Zen monks and those who have practiced meditation for many years. All I can say is that one really needs to experience a float to fully understand it.

What is Floatation Therapy?

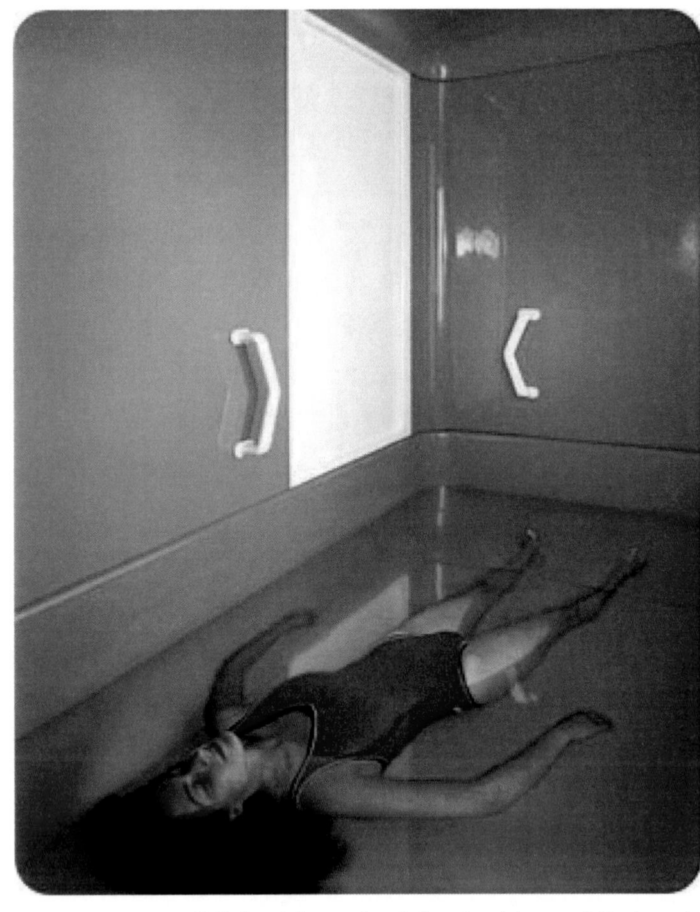

In a nutshell, floatation therapy is a method by which one can easily obtain the deepest physical and mental rest and relaxation very quickly. Essentially, it's spending hour or so floating quietly in a purpose-built float tank containing a highly concentrated Epsom salts solution, twelve inches deep and so dense that you float effortlessly. The solution is heated to 35 degrees Celsius to match your body's skin temperature for maximum comfort.

The dimensions of the float tank installed at my health centre measure 8.5 feet long by 4 foot wide and it stands 7 foot tall. This allows ample space inside to move around and stretch out and also, to lessen any claustrophobic worries.

(see: www.naturaltherapy.ie/floatation-tanks.html).

The Float

Unless you happen to be an astronaut, floating in water is the only time that your body is going to be free of the forces of gravity and this in itself is a quite extraordinary feeling. The combination of weightlessness and the absence of external stimuli enable the body to relax deeply. In this zero gravity environment all your muscles will relax simultaneously while your brain enters a deep "Theta" meditative-like state, much akin to being hypnotised.

Floating does not require any swimming skills, as you actually float like a cork, no matter what weight or shape you are. Your skin will not wrinkle either; due to the high salt content of the water (wrinkling is actually caused by water leaching salts from your skin).

During the float there should be no feelings of being confined in a tight space. The lights and door are controlled by you so even if you are feeling claustrophobic, you can choose to float with the light on and the door open. You are always in total control. You just need a willingness on your part to let go and see what happens. During the float you can also choose to hear gentle music in the tank to further help you relax.

Some people may need to float a few times before they are able to completely relax both mentally and physically. Generally though, one quickly enters a profoundly relaxed state where they will lose all sense of time and drift off into a dream-like state, partially induced by the release of endorphins, the body's feel-good chemicals. After your floatation session ends, this euphoric feeling will stay with you for many hours and even days. And the more often you float, the better it gets. People who regularly float experience a raft of health benefits most of which are listed below.

The Health Benefits of Floating

Apart from general relaxation research has shown floatation therapy to measurably reduce blood pressure and heart rate whilst also lowering the levels of the stress hormone cortisol in the body. In addition, endorphins, the body's natural opiates and painkillers are released.

As you relax in the warm salt solution, your capillaries and larger blood vessels all dilate, increasing blood flow and facilitating the elimination of metabolic wastes and other toxins from your body. This benefits arthritic pains, muscle spasms and tenderness; often eliminating the need for pain controlling drugs entirely. For example, individuals suffering from the constant pain of fibromyalgia, get amazing relief when regularly taking floats.

But floating isn't just for people in pain. As a society, most people in this day and age are under enormous mental pressure in their daily lives and so: a one hour floatation session, allows their brain and nervous system to power down and recuperate.

Floating is also helpful for insomnia (one hour float has the restorative effects of six hours of sleep), for fatigue, for mental concentration and creativity, and for detoxification (Epsom salts draws toxins out of the body).

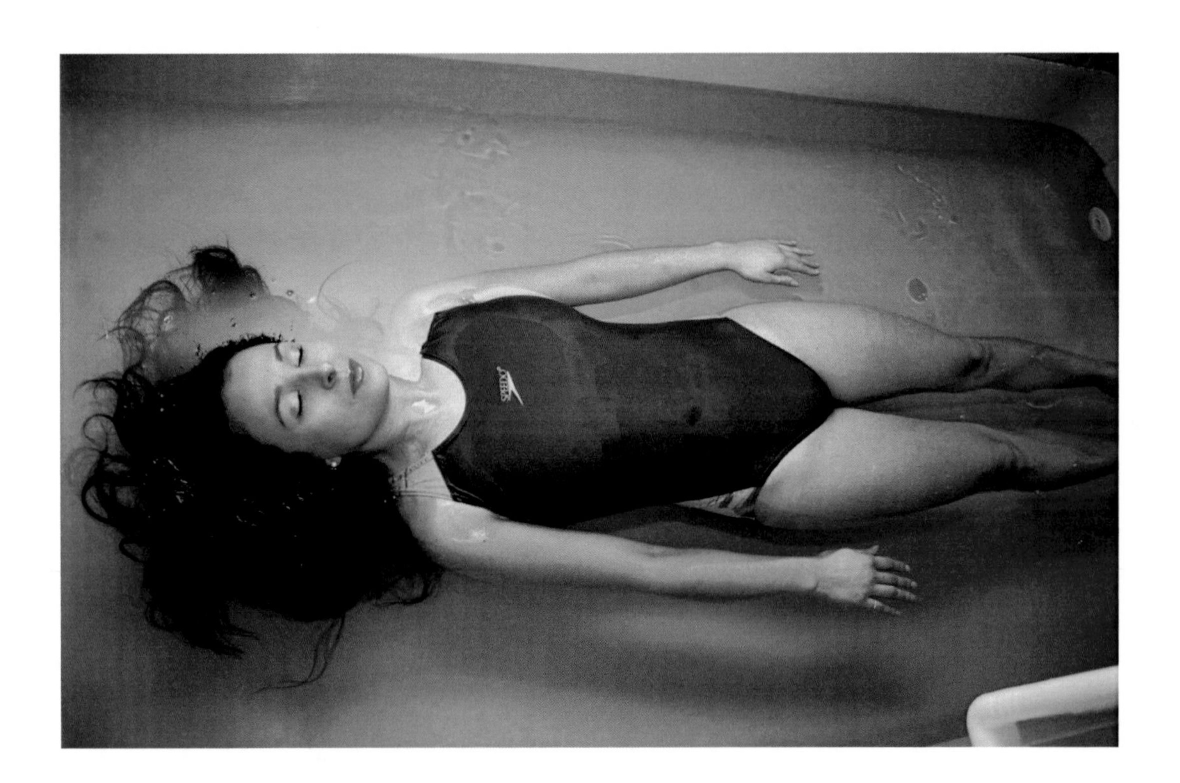

In a nutshell: Floating can help with the following:

- Intense physical and mental relaxation
- Relieves stress
- Lowers levels of the stress hormone cortisol
- Releases endorphins (body's feel-good hormone)
- Decreases anxiety
- Improves mental concentration
- Improves sleep patterns
- Increases energy levels
- Pain-relief from back injuries and muscle and joint pain
- Detoxification of the body
- Improves the condition of the skin
- Provides relief from aches and pains during pregnancy
- Increase creativity by balancing the left and right brain hemispheres.

Light Therapy

Light therapy has been documented in research literature for the past fifty years, to deliver powerful therapeutic healing benefits to body tissues. The studies have focussed on a specific type of light generated by a laser, known as 'Low-Level Laser Therapy' (LLLT).

The word **LASER** is actually an acronym for **Light Amplification by Stimulated Emission Radiation.** A laser generates a specific wavelength of light, not an entire spectrum, like a light bulb does. The beams of light generated by lasers are very concentrated and intense and are referred to as 'coherent' light whereas a light bulb generates diffuse light that is referred to as 'non-coherent' light.

There are two types of laser used by industry; 1) High power (hot) lasers and 2) Low energy (cold) lasers. High power lasers can cut through body tissues like a surgeon's scalpel, whereas low-level lasers (the type we'll be using) do not have a thermal component that can cause injuries to body tissues. The reason being, when the light energy from a low-level laser hits the skin, it scatters and dissipates over a wider surface area, providing safe and gentle, yet powerful healing benefits.

The mechanisms by which light therapy causes positive biological effects on the body's tissues are complex, but essentially rely upon the absorption of specific wavelengths of light, by photoreceptors within the mitochondria of cells. If you can remember back to studying biology at school when you learned about photosynthesis in plants, remember how chlorophyll traps light energy from the sun and converts it to adenosine triphosphate (ATP) by cellular respiration. (ATP is the fuel of all living cells whether plant or animal).

Similarly, in human cells Low-Level Laser light energy can stimulate the photoreceptor 'cytochrome-C-oxidase' in the mitochondria of the cell to increase ATP production. This increases cellular metabolism and as a result our cells repair faster and survive longer. Dr. Harry T. Whelan of the Medical College of Wisconsin conducted many studies on light therapy on behalf of NASA, and these studies have demonstrated that when cells are exposed to low-level light therapy, they exhibit a massive increase in cellular metabolism suggesting enhanced cellular repair and vitality.(43)

Numerous other studies over the past fifty years have also shown light therapy to influence as much as 24 positive changes within the body at cellular level including:

- Stimulates the production of ATP (energy currency for a cell), which increases cellular metabolism
- Down-regulates the inflammatory response, decreasing inflammation and speeding up the healing process.
- Promotes cell repair and cell regeneration.
- Stimulates the production and release of nitric oxide from haemoglobin and surrounding tissues. (Nitric oxide relaxes smooth muscles that are abundant in blood vessel walls and lymphatic vessels. These vessels will then dilate, increasing circulation and the consequent elimination of the body's

metabolic end- wastes).

- Nitric oxide is also a neurotransmitter in the brain (neurotransmitters are chemicals that relay electrical messages from one nerve cell to another).
- Relieves pain in body tissues by reducing the synthesis of pro-inflammatory proteins and by the rapid regeneration of damaged nerve fibres.
- Stimulates the production of collagen, the most abundant protein in the body and essential for the repair of damaged tissue. By increasing collagen production, less scar tissue is formed at the damaged site.
- Speeds up the healing of bone fractures and increases bone density reversing osteoporosis.

The Light Therapy device I use at my clinic is called the **'Avalon Light Therapy System'**. It uses Light Emitting Diodes (LEDs) that generate specific wavelengths of light, pulsed at research proven frequencies. Pulsed light has been shown to be more effective than non-pulsed light, and those pulsed to body tissue resonance frequencies are the most effective in the healing response.

LEDs are similar to low-level lasers in the healing response; however they disperse light over a greater surface area, which results in a shorter treatment time.

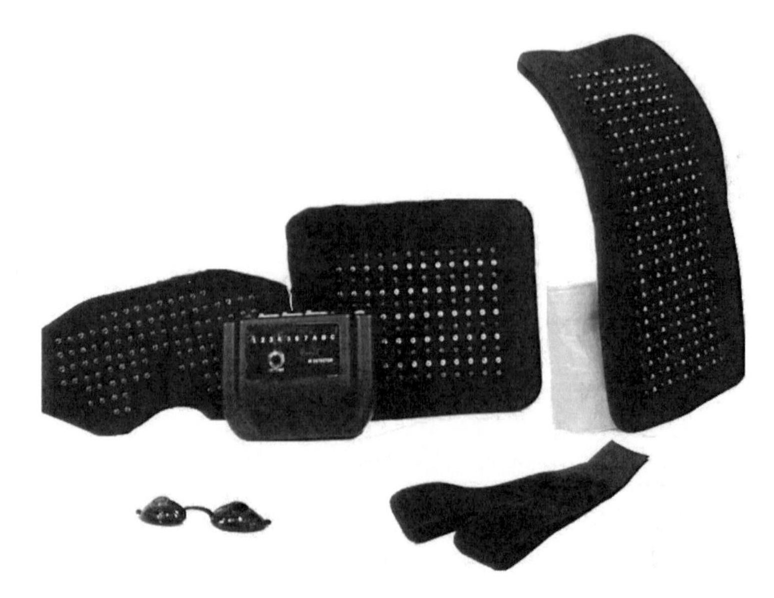

The wavelengths of light generated by the Avalon

device have frequencies of 440, 640 and 880 nanometres, corresponding to the colours red, blue and infrared (invisible to humans) respectively. Research has shown these frequencies to have the best biological effects on human tissue. For instance:

Red Light –which does not penetrate as deeply as infrared, seems to help wounds heal more quickly. In addition, the light can be used to remove certain precancerous skin cells without scarring according to David Goldberg, M.D., director of Skin Laser & Surgery Specialists of New York & New Jersey. Red light promotes collagen formation, which smooth out wrinkles. Red light also has an anti-inflammatory effect and can kill bacteria, as can blue light. In fact, using red and blue light together can be very effective in treating severe cases of acne.

Blue Light – Besides its use as an antibacterial agent, blue light has a special ability to reset the biological clock. Studies indicate "blue light boxes" are far more effective than full-spectrum sunlight boxes of equal intensity at fighting seasonal affective disorder, commonly known as SAD or the winter blues. Other studies at Harvard Medical School in Boston also indicate that a dose of blue light, depending on when it is given, can increase alertness or help fight insomnia.(44) So, blue frequencies are best for treatments of skin, anti-aging, rejuvenation and moods.

Infra-red light – with its long wavelengths can penetrate deeply into human tissue, bringing healing at deeper levels by reducing pain and inflammation in deep muscles, bones and joints.

The **Avalon Light Therapy System** can also reduce stress and emotional blockages in the body via an inbuilt compilation of Quantum, Salfeggio, Schumann and Nogier frequencies, for the most desirable healing results.

I have been using the Avalon light therapy system on my clients for the past three years and have had nothing but positive feedback from everyone. They experience everything from a more relaxed state of mind, to skin healing (i.e. skin ulcers and cellulitis), to pain relief, to muscle relaxation and to more joint flexibility.

Chapter 8

SUPPORT FOR THE NERVOUS SYSTEM

> An intact nervous system will lead to optimum functioning of the human body

The nervous system is the first body system to develop in the human embryo – an indication of its importance to the rest of the body. The nervous system is the predominant co-ordinator of all body functions; from the respiration of a single cell to the regulatory effect it exerts over all major body systems. All levels of health, including the mental, emotional and physical are influenced by the condition of the nervous system.

Proper functioning of your nervous system relies upon a number of factors including adequate nutrients obtained from your diet. It is one of the systems most likely to suffer imbalance as a result of poor nutrition, environmental toxins and lifestyle habits. Nutritional and also herbal support is tremendously important for good nervous system health, especially considering the typical onslaught of junk foods, which the body must contend with in today's diet.

Nervous System Overview

The nervous system is divided into two principal divisions:

1. The Central Nervous System (CNS), which consists of the brain and the spinal cord.

2. The Peripheral Nervous System (PNS), which consists of the spinal nerves that emerge from the spinal cord and the cranial nerves that arise from the brain.

Despite the complexity of the nervous system it consists of only two principal kinds of cells: **neurons** and **neuroglia.**

Neurons are responsible for most functions attributed to the nervous system such as movement, breathing, heartbeat, sensing, thinking, memory and the regulation of glandular secretions.

Neuroglias functions are to support, nurture and protect the neurons

The Brain The adult brain is an irregular globe of moist gelatinous grey tissue containing around 100 billon neurons and many more neuroglia. Each neuron can be connected to thousands of other neurons via connections called synapses. Synaptic connections have small gaps, much like the gaps in a car's spark plug and it's across this space that chemical messengers called neurotransmitters are released.

Each neuron consists of a central body called the nerve cell and extending from it are its processes, which are called axons and dendrites. Axons relay the messages away from the nerve cell and the dendrites carry the message to the cell. Nerves have only one axon but many dentrites (see illustration).

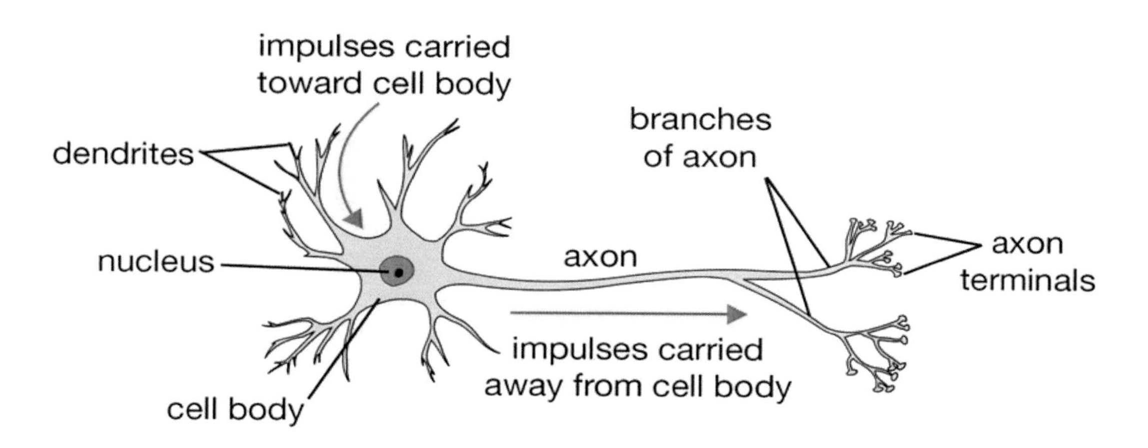

Many axons have a sleeve of fatty material that surrounds them called the myelin sheath – a type of insulation that allows for efficient nerve signal transmission. Made up of a range of proteins and fats (called lipoproteins), myelin surrounds, insulates and protects nerve axons helping to increase the rate at which nerves can transmit signals. Damage to or loss of myelin can prevent proper nerve signalling leading one to experience any number of symptoms of nerve dysfunction, common ones being pins and needles, muscle weakness, nerve pain and diminished vision.

> An extreme example of the damaging effects of myelin sheath degeneration is seen in patients who suffer from the condition, Multiple Sclerosis (MS). The signs and symptoms observed in these individuals' results from the progressive destruction of myelin, which slows and short-circuits conduction of nerve impulses. The result is a progressive loss of function in motor skills leading to immobility.

The axon of a neuron breaks into a cluster of small branches at its end, each branch terminating in small swellings called synaptic end-bulbs. These end-bulbs are in close proximity to the dendrites and cell body of adjoining neurons. When the nerve impulses reach the end-bulbs, a chemical substance is released, which stimulates the adjoining neuron into activity. Thus "charged" the adjoining neurons fire their own chemicals and this activity is repeated many millions of times in the brain and throughout the nervous system each second of our lives.

These chemical substances are called neurotransmitters and to date more than 100 different types have been identified. As soon as the neurotransmitter has stimulated the next neuron, it is immediately neutralised by an enzyme and made inactive, otherwise your nerves would be constantly over firing. Think of anyone suffering from an epilepsy fit!

Movement, thinking, memory, moods, appetite, sex drive and a number of other cognitive processes are controlled by your neurotransmitters, which also puts you to sleep, wakes you up and make you tense or happy.

Most neurotransmitters are made from amino acids obtained from the protein in your diet. Two of the most important neurotransmitters are serotonin and dopamine, commonly known as the "happy" molecules. Serotonin is synthesized from the amino acid tryptophan and dopamine is derived from the phenylalamine family of amino acids. The synthesis of both neurotransmitters also relies heavily on the presence of a number of nutrients including the B-vitamins and specific minerals in order to be properly synthesized by enzymes in the brain. Deficiencies in any of these nutrients can impede your body's ability to synthesize these neurotransmitters and in turn interfere with communication within your nervous system.

Signs and Symptoms of a Stressed Nervous System

If you're not getting a sufficient amount of the nutrients needed for good nervous system health, you may experience a range of symptoms from physical to psychological. As your nervous system is active right throughout your body, from your brain to the tips of your fingers and toes many symptoms in many areas of the body can be related to disorders with the nervous system. Some of the most common physical and psychological symptoms associated with disorders of the nervous system are:

- Pins and needles sensation anywhere in the body
- Loss of strength in the grip
- Poor co-ordination or abnormally accident prone
- Ringing or buzzing in the ears (tinnitus)
- Lightheaded or dizziness

- Loss of feeling or numbness in the extremities
- Heavy feeling in the limbs
- Heavy feeling in the head
- Burning feet
- Muscle cramps or nervous twitches
- Fatigue or exhaustion on the slightest effort
- Anxiety, depression and irritability
- Insomnia

Support for the Nervous System

Diet: One of the easiest things you can do to help ensure a healthy nervous system is to eat the right kinds of food containing high levels of all the nutrients essential to supporting and nourishing nerve tissue and proper nerve function. Following is a brief overview of several nutrients that play a key role in keeping your nervous system healthy and working the way it should.

The B Vitamins

The B-complex vitamins are very important for overall nervous system health. Often referred to, as the "stress" vitamins, due to their physiological uses for improving the body's natural stress coping mechanisms, any deficiencies in one or more of these water-soluble vitamins will quickly result in both physical and psychological symptoms, as earlier described. The synthesis of neurotransmitters rely on the presence of these B vitamins especially vitamins B1, B3, B5, B6, B9 and B12. Because they are water-soluble these vitamins are quickly excreted out of the body and therefore are required in sufficient amounts on a daily basis. As the modern diet is generally insufficient in supplying the requisite amounts of vitamins and minerals for the body's needs (see chapter 9), any nutritional programme targeting the nervous system should include a high quality vitamin B-complex.

Vitamin B1 (Thiamine)

Vitamin B1 is required for glucose metabolism, glucose being the primary fuel for the brain. A deficiency of this vitamin first manifests as physical and mental fatigue. A chronic deficiency of B1 can lead to nerve damage manifesting as a burning sensation in the limbs, as well as pins and needles sensation in the hands and feet. The disease beriberi, which affects the nerves to the limbs, producing pain, paralysis and swelling is caused by a prolonged deficiency in thiamine.

Foods high in thiamine include whole grains, eggs, liver, brewer's yeast, beans, green leaf vegetables and sunflower seeds.

Vitamin B3 (Niacin)

Vitamin B3 deficiencies have been associated with mental and personality disorders. The most well-known symptoms of a chronic B3 deficiency is the disease Pellagra, characterised by the 4D's: Dermatitis, Diarrhoea, Dementia and Death. Vitamin B3 is essential in all living cells as a component of the co-enzymes NAD and NADP, and so is needed for nervous tissue and repair.

Foods high in vitamin B3 include: chicken, beef, liver, eggs, whole milk, spinach and peanut butter.

Vitamin B5 (Pantothenic acid)

Vitamin B5 is needed for adrenal support and for the production of acetylcholine, the neurotransmitter associated with memory. Deficiency signs are very general due to the central role in metabolism. However, some signs and symptoms related to the nervous system may include fatigue, irritability, disturbed sleep, headache, shooting pains, muscle weakness and burning feet.

The best food sources of vitamin B5 are whole grains, legumes, brewer's yeast, salmon, calf liver, mushrooms, broccoli, cauliflower and royal jelly.

Vitamin B6 (Pyridoxine)

Vitamin B6 is needed for the production of serotonin and dopamine, two important neurotransmitters involved in nerve-cell communication. Prolonged deficiency of B6 can mimic all the signs of vitamin B3 deficiency and some of the signs of vitamin B5 deficiency.

On occasion I have prescribed high doses of vitamin B6 along with a B-complex to relieve numbness and tingling in the hands, cramping and spasms, swelling and weakness of the hands and poor co-ordination.

Good dietary sources of vitamin B6 include brewer's yeast, bananas, potatoes, sunflower seeds, chickpeas and wheat germ.

Vitamin B9 (Folic acid or Folate)

Vitamin B9, commonly called folic acid, along with vitamins B3, B6 and B12 are involved in methylation reactions. Such reactions are central to the formation of neurotransmitters. Folic acid is found in high amounts in the cerebral spinal fluid. It has long been observed that low levels of B9 in the body are associated with mental health problems such as depression and dementia. Other symptoms include mental sluggishness, irritability and restless leg syndrome. According to the WHO in Geneva, deficiency of vitamin B9 is widespread, especially in pregnant women and those on a low vegetable diet. Pregnant women are encouraged to take folic acid supplements to prevent spina bifida, a neural tube defect, in their newborns.

Foods high vitamin B9 include green leafy vegetables, citrus fruits, legumes, avocados, sunflower seeds, peanuts, brewer's yeast, liver and egg yolk.

Vitamin B12 (Cobalamin)

Vitamin B12 is essential for proper nerve functioning by helping to maintain healthy myelin, the nerve insulator that allows for good nerve transmission. B12 is also involved in the manufacture of methyl groups needed for methylation reactions in the production of neurotransmitters. B12 also helps break complex carbohydrates into glucose, the sugar your brain uses as fuel to carry out its functions.

A vitamin B12 deficiency can cause symptoms such as numbness and tingling in the hands and feet as a result of inflammation and demyelination of the nerves. Other symptoms can include poor muscle co-ordination, weakness in the legs, poor memory and confusion.

Foods rich in vitamin B12 include shellfish, salmon, mackerel, sardines, tuna, red meat, liver, poultry, eggs and dairy products. Foods derived from plants do not contain vitamin B12, so vegans need to acquire it from fermented foods, seaweeds and brewer's yeast as well as by supplementation.

Vitamin C (Ascorbic acid)

Not only is vitamin C important for good immune health along with a host of other biological functions in the body, it also plays an important role in the nervous system. It is involved in making the neurotransmitters noradrenaline and serotonin, which affect mood and wellbeing. Additionally it helps build collagen, the elastic tissue that keeps blood vessels flexible for improved blood flow to your brain. It is also an excellent antioxidant and so helps prevent the build-up of pro-inflammatory toxins and body wastes that can otherwise damage the nervous system.

Good food sources of vitamin C include citrus fruits and most vegetables.

Potassium and Sodium

These two minerals play an important role in nerve transmission by regulating the nerve impulses. Specifically, they make up the electrochemical signals that transmit nerve impulses throughout the cell. Over the duration of the nerve impulse sodium and potassium ions flood into and out of the neurons thus creating weak electrical signals throughout the nerve axon. Deficiencies in either of these minerals can adversely affect nerve signalling, causing both the brain and peripheral nervous system to malfunction.

Eating foods rich in potassium like bananas, sweet potatoes, white beans, tomato-based foods, yoghurt and clams as well as consuming small amounts of sea salt will ensure adequate levels of these two important minerals remain in your body to support proper nerve functioning.

Calcium and Magnesium

Similar to sodium and potassium, the minerals calcium and magnesium are also very important for maintaining the correct signals in the nervous system. Calcium helps initiate a nerve impulse and magnesium helps return the nerve to its resting state after the signal has been transmitted. Both of these minerals work hand in hand and a deficiency of either one will leave you more prone to muscle cramping, irritable and moody, and unable to sleep.

Foods rich in calcium include dairy products, seafood, sesame seeds, beans and green vegetables. Dark green leafy vegetables are high in magnesium due to it being a component of the molecule chlorophyll that gives plants their green colour. Other foods high in magnesium are nuts and seeds such as pumpkin, sunflower, sesame and cashews.

Essential Fatty Acids (omega-3 and omega-6)

Essential Fatty Acids (EFA's) benefit every cell in the body including nerve cells. They are part of the lipid-rich membrane structure that surrounds cells and keeps them intact. They help make up the myelin sheath that covers nerve axons. They are also precursors for the production of prostaglandins – extremely active hormone-like substances that regulate the release and performance of neurotransmitters in the brain and nervous system.

Often referred to as "brain food", these two essential fatty acids have been demonstrated to help improve intelligence and behavioural problems in children as well as help individuals suffering from depression and other mental conditions.

Foods high in omega-3 fats include oily fish such as salmon, mackerel, herring, sardines, tuna and anchovies; seeds such as chia-bia, pumpkin and flaxseed along with walnuts. Omega-6 rich foods include seeds such as sunflower, sesame, safflower and pumpkin as well as eggs, whole grains and most vegetable oils.

As I explained earlier in chapter 2, the balance of omega-3 to omega-6 fatty acid intake in our modern Western diet is skewed heavily in favour of omega-6 by a ratio of roughly 20:1. This ratio should ideally be closer to 2:1. One therefore should try to focus on consuming more omega-3 rich foods.

Phospholipids

Phospholipids are a special class of fats that make up cell membranes – the skin that surrounds every living cell in the body. As the name implies phospholipids are composed of a phosphate group of atoms attached to two fatty acids called EPA and DHA that are made from omega-3 fatty acids.

Phospholipids form a lipid bi-layer membrane that allows for membrane fluidity while also controlling what flows in and out of each cell. These specialised lipids are an integral part in the make-up of the myelin sheath that covers nerve axons and so are critically important to the proper transmission of nerve signals. Phospholipids are also needed to make acetylcholine, the neurotransmitter involved in memory. They are also a component of prostaglandins – a class of biochemically active substances that help regulate neurotransmitters. In addition, phospholipids supply nutrients for the methylation pathways, which are critical to the smooth running of the body's neurotransmitters.

Phospholipids possess many pro-health properties including acting neuro-protectively on the nervous system, regulation of brain activity, enhances memory recall and increases resistance to stress. Supplemental use has proven helpful in the treatment of Alzheimer's disease and manic depression.

The body naturally produces phospholipids; however, consuming phospholipid-rich food sources can boost their health-giving presence in the body. One of the most plentiful sources of phospholipids is lecithin, which appears naturally in foods such as egg yolk, soya beans, sunflower seeds, peanuts, wheat germ, milk, sardines and caviar (fish eggs).

Lecithin is composed of a mixture of phospholipids, notably choline and inositol. Choline is used in the manufacture of acetylcholine, the neurotransmitter associated with memory. Lecithin is widely available in health food shops as a supplement, usually in granule form. A heaped dessertspoonful of it sprinkled over your cereal in the morning will provide you with ample amounts of this health-enhancing supplement. It can also be taken in yoghurts or mixed in smoothes.

Protein

Most neurotransmitters are made from amino acids obtained from the protein in food you consume. Dopamine, the "happy" neurotransmitter is made from the amino acid tyrosine. Once produced, dopamine can in turn be converted into noradrenaline and adrenaline. Low levels of dopamine can cause you to feel depressed, lethargic and withdrawn. Without going into detailed brain chemistry, small amounts (100 – 150grams) of protein-rich food will elevate dopamine levels within 30 minutes of ingestion, increasing alertness and energy levels. High protein foods include fish, meat, poultry, eggs and legumes.

Tyrosine is also needed in forming the nerve chemical and adrenal hormone adrenaline and it may improve memory or mood in people when they are under stress. Sources include lean meat, eggs, milk, and soya foods.

Serotonin is made from the essential amino acid tryptophan (essential meaning that it needs to come from the diet). Also known as the "happy" molecule, this neurotransmitter is important to feelings of wellbeing and contentment. Low levels of serotonin can induce feelings of anger, anxiety and depression, so consuming foods high in tryptophan such as turkey can counteract these negative feelings. Other food sources high in tryptophan include cheese, oily fish, eggs, milk, sesame seeds, pumpkin seeds, legumes and dark chocolate.

L-glutamine, a non-essential amino acid (meaning your body can manufacture it) is the precursor to gamma-amino butyric acid (GABA), the neurotransmitter that helps regulate the nervous system and promote calmness. Once L-glutamine is converted into GABA it acts as an antidepressant having a sedative effect and improving sleep.

L-glutamine can also be used as an alternative energy source by brain cells, increasing alertness, memory and sustained concentration – great for exam study. While your body normally makes all the glutamine it needs, situations like a prolonged illness may require you to increase your dietary intake by eating more protein-rich foods such as meat, fish, poultry, eggs and dairy products like cottage cheese and whey.

Herbal Support for the Nervous System

Nowhere is the efficacy of herbal medicine more evident than in problems related to the nervous system. Most chronic diseases have an etiological component of nervous system imbalance caused by poor diet and various lifestyle factors. Whilst it's important to address all the underlying factors leading to ill health, particular attention needs to be given to supporting nerve function. In my consultations I always include herbal medicines that feed and nourish nerve tissue to restore proper nerve function.

Nervine tonics, also known as **adaptogens** or **tropho-restoratives** are a class of herbal medicines that possess normalising and rejuvenating qualities. They act to nourish, strengthen and heal nerve tissue, restoring tone and function to the nervous system. They are therapeutically effective for both overactive and underactive functional states of the nervous system including:

- Nervous debility and exhaustion
- Depression
- Nervous tension
- Anxiety

The therapeutic effects of nervine tonic herbs are witnessed over a period of some weeks to months as they work to provide improvement in the tone and function of the nervous system.

Some examples of the great herbal restoratives of the nervous system are Avena sativa (Oats), Bacopa monniera (Bacopa), Scutellaria lateriflora (Scullcap), Eleutherococcus senticosus (Siberian Ginseng), Turnera diffusa (Damiana) and Withania somnifera (Ashwaganda)

Avena sativa (Oats)

Avena Sativa is an excellent nutritive herb and nerve tonic containing high amounts of B vitamins and other nutrients essential for proper functioning of the nervous system. It is a rich source of protein and contains a number of important minerals, lipids and fibre. Avena has a wide spectrum of biological activities within the body where it works not only physically but also psychologically, strengthening, feeding and revitalising the nervous system.

Bacopa monniera (Bacopa)

Bacopa monniera, also called Brahmi, originates from India – is well known for its benefits to the brain. Research shows that its active ingredients, nitric oxide and the fatty acid B-sitostrol, have powerful and positive effects on learning and memory recall. Studies confirm that adults who took bacopa daily have better short-term memories than those who took a placebo. While supporting our intelligence, this powerful herb can improve our capacity to focus and withstand emotional stress. I often use bacopa for students and for those clients suffering considerable stress.

Scutellaria lateriflora (Scullcap)

Scutellaria lateriflora has the double action of relaxing nervous tension while also nourishing and supporting the central nervous system. It is useful in conditions of nervous tension, nervous exhaustion and debility. As a mild bitter it will also help stimulate digestion and help the liver.

Eleutherococcus senticosus (Siberian Ginseng)

Eleutherococcus is an "adaptogen" that helps to balance the entire system. Chinese herbalists call it "The King of the Adaptogens". It gives strength and fortitude, especially when dealing with stress; so often a factor in illness. Patients complaining of mild health disturbances including exhaustion, irritability, insomnia and mild depression respond well to a course of eleutherococcus. I've used eleutherococcus on a regular basis for 20 years and I've recommended it to hundreds of patients. Eleutherococcus is a safe and invaluable addition to any nutritional regimen.

Turnera diffusa (Damiana)

Turnera diffusa is a nervine herb with tonic and trophorestorative properties. It has long been used as an aphrodisiac to boost sexual potency by the indigenous tribes of South America. It is indicated for treatment of sexual problems as well as for boosting and maintaining mental and physical stamina. Turnera diffusa can also be used to relieve anxiety, nervousness, and mild depression, especially if these symptoms have a sexual component.

Withania somnifera (Ashwaganda)

Withania somnifera is a rejuvenative tonic herb. It is the most frequently prescribed tonic in Ayurvedic medicine. It is able to increase energy and endurance.

It promotes longevity, supports sexual vitality, calms the mind, enhances mental functioning, rejuvenates the body's tissues, strengthens the immune system, improves sleep, and helps the body to overcome any imbalances that may have been caused by stress, poor diet and lack of sleep or environmental factors.

But the list does not stop here. Some other notable examples of adaptogen herbs include **Rosmarinus officinalis (Rosemary),** which helps the circulation to the brain, strengthens mental clarity and is therefore useful in geriatric senility.

Ginkgo biloba also promotes circulation to the brain. There is even growing evidence that Ginkgo can help in the fight against Alzheimer's disease and dementia, possibly because of its benefits for circulation to the brain. Ginkgo is a 'Prescription Only' herb, which can only be obtained from a reputable herbalist.

Gotu Kola *(Centella asiatica)*, can improve brain function by improving blood flow and memory. It has been used for centuries in Ayurvedic medicine as a nerve tonic and to treat insomnia, stress, anxiety and memory problems.

St. John's Wort *(Hypericum perforatum)*, used for a range of nerve disorders, it has become one of the most popular herbs due to its use as a mild to moderate antidepressant. It works by raising the levels of serotonin in the brain and needs 2 to 4 weeks to develop its mood elevating effects. Like Ginkgo, it too is a 'Prescription Only' herb; and while it is considered to be safe with no apparent side-effects, it should not be taken with other psychoactive drugs.

Of course, the choice of a nervine herb most suitable to an individual patient must be based upon a thorough health assessment and the experience and training of a qualified naturopath/herbal practitioner. But even the layperson can do much to alleviate stress and soothe frayed nerves. Drinking herbal teas like chamomile, lemon balm and valerian is the sensible choice instead of coffee for anyone having sleeping difficulties or anyone who wishes to achieve a deeper sense of inner calm.

"ODYLIRESIN" – SWISS FORMULA FOOD SUPPLEMENT

An Herbal Adaptogen in a class all of its own!

If ever there was a plant extract capable of increasing the body's ability to resist the damaging effects of stress and that can restore normal physiological functioning, it has to be "ODYLIRESIN".

ODYLIRESIN is an herbal formula of ***Iresine celosia,*** a plant from Central America, belonging to the family Amaranthacae. This herb is rich in substances such as glucocorticoids, various natural proteins, flavonoids, pectins and anti-oxidants, which have been shown to affect neuro-endocrine glandular secretions, improve defence mechanisms of the body, and to promote both physical and mental health in those taking it.

First discovered in 1960 by the eminent naturopath, Efrain Contreras (1898 – 1986), he studied its therapeutic virtues and found it useful for treating a wide variety of medical conditions, most notably cancer. Other researchers have later demonstrated how Iresine celosia, given in therapeutic doses affects the permeability of cancer cell membranes by changing their bio-electrical properties, and also by enhancing the transcription of tumour suppressor proteins.

Its clinical uses can be described as "full-spectrum". I take a few drops of ODYLIRESIN under my tongue twice daily as a prophylactic. However, since I started taking it, I've noticed my concentration levels have greatly improved and in the mornings when I wake up, I want to jump straight out of bed just like my two young children do!

CHAPTER 9

THE QUESTION OF NUTRIENT SUPPLEMENTATION

> *"Nearly all disease can be traced to a nutritional deficiency"*
> *- Dr. Linus Pauling*

The need to supplement one's diet with vitamins and minerals has always been a contentious issue with most doctors and dieticians of the opinion that if you eat a well- balanced diet, it will provide you with all the vitamins and minerals along with other micro-nutrients necessary for good health, therefore it is foolish to take supplements.

Maybe this may have been possible 50 to 100 years ago when food was grown organically on fertile soils and was not stripped of its nutrients through any refining and packaging process and so contained all the nutrients that nature intended.

But today the choice to eat a well-balanced diet is no longer within our control. Ideally, we should be able to get all of our nutrients from natural food sources, but unfortunately the nutritional value of today's modern diet is inadequate to meet even the basic requirements for maintaining optimal health. That's because so many of the foods available today have been stripped of much of their nutrient content through over-processing and refining techniques.

> Nutrient supplementation may be defined as the deliberate addition of nutrients (i.e. vitamins, minerals, amino acids, essential fatty acids or probiotics) to the diet with the intention of preventing or correcting possible nutrient deficiencies, preventing or curing particular diseases and/or optimising overall health.

In addition, due to intensive farming practices, our soils have become depleted of minerals essential for human health.

In fact, as far back as 1936, a U.S. Senate Document [#264report] stated that the soil was so nutritionally deficient of minerals that it would not supply the necessary nutrition for good health.(45) This problem is not just confined to the U.S. A 1992 RIO Earth Summit report concluded *"There is deep concern over continuing major declines in the mineral values in farm and range soils throughout the world".* This statement was based on data showing that over the last 100 years, average mineral levels in agricultural soils has fallen worldwide – by 72% in Europe, 76% in Asia and 85% in North America. Considering the fact that this report was published over 22 years ago, the soil would now be even worse since to this day nothing has been done to rectify it.

Only three of the necessary 60 minerals the body needs, are put back into the soil in intensive agricultural practices – nitrogen, potassium and phosphorus, which are the only minerals plants require for growth. Although these crops appear luscious the foods derived from them are nutrient-deficient. Then, to compound matters even more, if there is too much nitrates in the soil, it will prevent the absorption of other minerals by the crops even if such minerals are present in sufficient quantities.

Also, the food crops growing on these depleted soils are loaded with residues of herbicides, pesticides and other chemical pollutants. The majority of fruits and vegetables are either sprayed or dipped in more chemicals at harvest time and then left in cold storage for long periods further depleting their nutrient content. Consequently, most food that arrives on our tables has very little in the way of vitamins, minerals or other micro-nutrients essential to human health.

According to Dr. Joel Wallach, a pioneering researcher in clinical nutrition who has spent half a century identifying and treating the underlying causes of disease, contends that the human body needs 90 essential nutrients to remain in optimum health.(46) These nutrients include:

- 60 minerals

- 16 vitamins
- 12 amino acids
- 2 essential fatty acids (A nutrient is called essential if the human body cannot make it).

If there are any deficiencies in one or more of these nutrients at their appropriate levels, deemed necessary for health, the body will malfunction and over time will develop some form of disease. According to Wallach, replenishing the body with the deficient nutrients will eliminate the diseases caused by such deficiencies. He also claims that it is simply impossible to get all 90 of these nutrients from our food supply today hence the need for supplementation.

This is backed up by governmental studies showing that the soil food is grown in is deficient in many essential minerals, and also multiple surveys have shown that the average person's diet is below the **Recommended Dietary Allowance (RDA)** in several different nutrients. The RDA's are a measure of the minimum amounts of the essential nutrients required by the body to maintain metabolic balance, or in other words, to prevent the development of a vitamin or mineral deficiency disease. They were calculated based upon the minimum amounts of nutrients needed to eliminate diseases like scurvy (a vitamin C deficiency), beriberi (a vitamin B1 deficiency), or pellagra (a vitamin B3 deficiency).

The governmental agencies responsible for determining the RDAs did not take into consideration that these calculated levels were never enough to prevent mild to moderate nutritional deficiencies the symptoms of which may often be subtle, overlapping and varied. For example, the first signs of vitamin B deficiency may include subtle changes in behaviours such as mood swings and an inability to concentrate and/or trouble falling asleep. Other signs and symptoms of nutritional deficiencies can include fatigue, anxiety, confusion, or muscle weakness. Even marginal deficiencies of vitamin B6 along with vitamins A, C, and E can reduce immunity, impairing the body's ability to ward off disease and repair damaged tissues.

Dr. Wallach contends that over 900 diseases are caused by deficiencies of the ninety essential nutrients. For example, he states that a simple calcium deficiency can cause any or all of the following conditions:

- High blood pressure
- Arthritis
- Osteoporosis
- Lower back pain
- Premenstrual syndrome (PMS)
- Tinnitus (ringing in the ears)
- Kidney stones
- Bell's palsy
- Trigeminal neuralgia
- Insomnia

Returning to the RDAs, there was also no consideration given for the great variability from person to person and that each individual's nutritional requirements are unique to that person. The RDAs were not calculated to take into account the nutrient requirements of anyone in ill health, the very young or old, pregnant women, athletes or those involved in strenuous occupations, obese people, smokers or those on medications, and so on......

So even if you were to meet all of the RDA guidelines, there is no way of knowing whether these amounts are specific for you, at your age and in your present state of health.

Nutrient requirements change constantly according to all sorts of demands. For example: an individual with a history of allergies requires amounts of vitamin B5 larger than what they could ever get from their diets. Or someone with a constitutional tendency to blood clotting or with a history of heart disease will benefit from a larger intake of vitamin E well above the RDA levels. A woman suffering from recurring premenstrual syndrome would need larger amounts of Vitamin B-Complex in addition to the minerals calcium and magnesium.

Then if we take into account the fact that there is nowhere we can go in the world today that is free from pollution and other environmental challenges, all this exposure to pollution along with the stress of modern living leads to an increased demand by the body for specific nutrients such as the antioxidant vitamins A, C and E along with the bioflavonoids and zinc above the RDA requirements and probably well above what most people obtain from their diet.

Also, consider on the off-chance that if you do consume highly nutritious foods that contain the recommended RDA levels, such foods may not be digested and absorbed properly by many people. So, the net result for such individuals is low blood and tissue levels of essential nutrients, causing derangement in body chemistry and thus setting the scene for disease. It is not just what we eat but what we absorb and utilise that matters.

When you consider that every bodily function totally depends on energy-producing chemical reactions taking place in the mitochondria (powerhouse) of our cells. These reactions produce ATP (our energy currency), which is then used by our cells to carry out their life-sustaining biochemical and metabolic functions. The amount of ATP produced depends on the availability of specific vitamins and minerals, and without adequate amounts of these nutrients together with the requisite carbohydrates, proteins and fats in our diet then energy is reduced at the cellular level, vitality diminishes and illness will occur.

So for optimum nutrition, the RDAs are simply not enough. So what is enough? Well, the work of Dr. Emanuel Cheraskin and his colleagues from the University of Alabama showed that the intake of nutrients associated with optimum health was often ten times or more higher than the RDA levels.(47) The levels shown in the table below and on the next page are deemed to be the daily amounts needed to maintain optimal health.

	Men		Women	
Nutrient	**RDA**	**SONA**	**RDA**	**SONA**
Fat-soluble Vitamins				
Vitamin A (RE, I RE = I micro gm = 3.33 IU)	1,000	2,000	800	2,000
Beta-carotene (mg)	N/A	100	N/A	80
Vitamin D (micro gm, 1 microgram = 40 IU)	5	24	5	24
Vitamin E (IU, 1 IU alpha tocopherol equivalent to I mg alpha tocopherol)	10	800	8	800
Vitamin K (mg)	80	80	65	65

Water-soluble Vitamins	**Men** RDA	SONA	**Women** RDA	SONA
Vitamin C (mg)	60	800	60	1000
Vitamin B12 (mg)	2	3	2	3
Folic acid (micro gm)	200	2000	180	2000
Niacin (mg)	15	30	15	25
Pyridoxine (B6) (mg)	2	25	1.6	20
Riboflavin (B 2) (mg)	1.4	2.5	1.2	2
Thiamin (B1) (mg)	1.2	9.2	1	9

Minerals	Men		Women	
	RDA	SONA	RDA	SONA
Boron (mg)	N/A	2.5	N/A	3
Calcium (mg)	800	700	800	1200
Chromium (micro gm)	50-200	300	50-200	300
Copper (mg)	1.5-3	1.5-4	1.5-3	1.5-4
Iodine (micro gm)	150	150	150	150
Iron (mg)	10	20	15	20
Magnesium (mg)	350	600	280	550
Manganese (mg)	2-5	10	2-5	10
Phosphorous (mg)	800	800	800	800
Potassium (mg)	99	200-500	99	200-500
Selenium (micro gm)	70	250	55	200
Sodium (mg)	500	400	500	400
Zinc (mg)	15	20	12	17

Dr Cheraskin came to these conclusions based on the efforts of a 15 year study to establish what he called a "**Suggested Optimum Nutrients Allowances**" or **SONA** for short.(47) These SONA levels are the levels of nutrients found in those people who participated in the study of 13, 500 male and female subjects who were relatively healthy as opposed to those with clinical symptoms and signs of disease.

A FEW SIMPLE CLUES FOR THE NEED FOR NUTRIENT SUPPLEMENTATION

Vitamin A....if your skin is bad, e.g. acne, gooseflesh, keratosis.

If your eyesight is poor, especially at night.

If any of the mucous membrane linings are inflamed; e.g. sinusitis, sore throats or lung problems, ulcers (both inside and outside), cystitis

Vitamin B....if you are tired and lethargic and 'not nice to be near'.

If you are irritable, even angry, your breath is bad, your feet, underarms and orifices are smelly you need B vitamins.

If you are stressed, especially if it is long term, you need vitamin B from every source you can get it. Burning feet can be a vitamin B5 deficiency.

If you have cracks and groves in your tongue (geographic tongue).

Vitamin C....if you bruise easily, if you have bleeding gums and loose teeth, if you suffer from dry eyes or floaters; if you have repeated infections; muscle spasms and muscle cramps.

Vitamin D...if you suffer from musculoskeletal pain or muscle fatigue, mood swings.

If you have osteopenia or osteoporosis, smoke and are overweight.

If you use sunscreens a lot, have heavily pigmented skin or live in Northern latitudes.

Vitamin E...if you have dry skin or if you are short of breath; if you suffer from poor circulation, mild anaemia, age spots, a decrease in sex drive, neurological pain, cataracts, dry hair or loss of hair.

Iron ....if you are tired, irritable and pale, you may need iron; a pale coloured nail-bed, spoon-shaped nails; pale lower eyelid (inside), bright red lines on stretched palms, or brittle hair.

Calcium.....if you are teary, irritable, suffer from restless legs, tinnitus (ringing in the ears), can't sleep at night, painful periods, have lower back pain or been diagnosed with osteoporosis. Other conditions that can be caused by low calcium levels include high blood pressure, kidney stones and Bell's palsy.

Children should have foods high in calcium and a calcium supplement in their major growth spurts.

Chromium.....if you have sugar cravings, if you suffer from blurred vision – like a film over the eye.

Magnesium..if you get muscle tics around the eye, muscle cramps, fatigue, dizziness, poor memory or confusion. If you have difficulty swallowing, have type 2 diabetes or suffer from poor heart health.

Zinc.............if you have white spots on your nails, have delayed wound healing, experience loss of either taste or smell, have stretch marks or get blisters between your fingers.

Omega-3 Fatty Acids...dry cracked skin on heels and fingertips, small bumps (like chicken skin) on the back of upper arms and legs; dry hair and dry eyes, dandruff, patches of pale skin on cheeks; build-up of ear wax, temper tantrums, depression or dementia; Attention Deficit, hyperactivity.

These are just a few simple clues that would prompt me to make the client aware of a deficiency or to add a supplement.

Ever since I've got into the natural health field, I've come across many sensationalistic news reports from outspoken critics of nutritional medicine pontificating on the potential dangers of vitamin and mineral supplement use. These assertions are usually based on studies carried out using cheap **low-grade synthetic vitamins and inorganic minerals.**

Synthetic vitamins are made in a laboratory where the chemist attempts to reconstruct the exact molecular structure of the nutrient in question. However, these man-made chemicals don't appear in nature. This is especially true of vitamin E, which in its synthetic form has the opposite molecular structure of vitamin E as found in nature.

This synthetic Vitamin E has already been used in different clinical trials, even though it is known to have a long history of being toxic for human consumption. Which begs the question: Are these pharmacological-supported trials intentionally designed to produce negative results?

Had these researchers bothered to test high-quality natural supplements instead of isolated synthetic ones, they would most likely have yielded more positive results for the subjects in their studies. The fact is: vitamins in their natural state always exist as living complexes with specific synergistic co-factors, enzymes, phytonutrients and organic minerals, and never as isolated single nutrients. A vitamin needs all of its synergists to function correctly.

It's my contention that these researchers are directed to test only isolated synthetic nutrients so as to use the negative results of the study to cast aspersion on all supplement use. What these trials really prove is only that synthetic chemical vitamins are toxic to human health. Such vitamins should more accurately be called **drugs!**

An image of crystallized Natural Vitamin E	*Synthetic Vitamin E; low electron energy levels make for less reflected light*

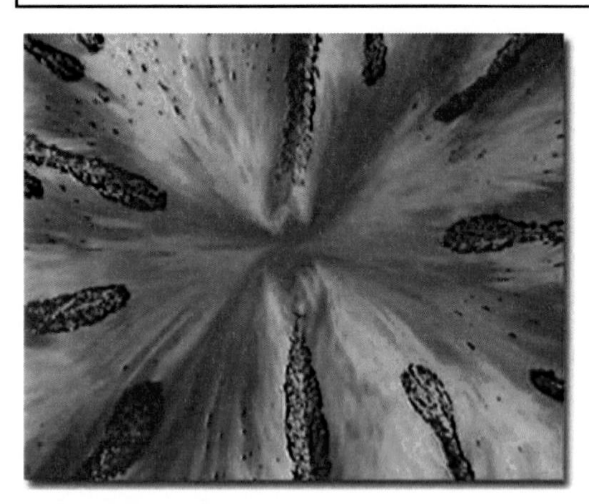

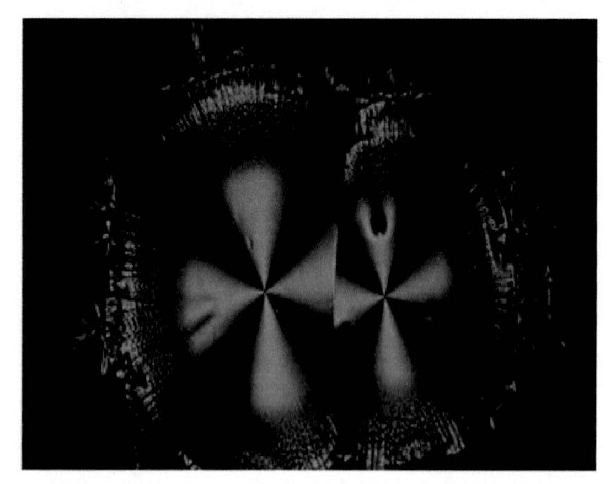

In natural vitamin E most of the outer electrons are in high quantum energy states, so they play with the light and make it shimmer. In synthetic vitamin E the electrons are in lower energy states and are photonic duds.

Then when the mainstream media report on these misleading studies, they gleefully claim that these supplements are worthless to human health, while utterly failing to differentiate between cheap synthetic-manufactured nutrients used in the studies versus high-quality food based natural nutrients. This, despite the fact that there is already an overwhelming amount of positive research in support of natural food-based supplements being able to support long term health and reduce the risk of many diseases.

My guess is, the real motivation behind all this junk science is to scare people away from using all nutritional supplements while at the same time brain-washing them into believing that they need vital pharmacological drugs and medical interventions in order to survive. That's the only pathway to health they would have you believe!

With natural supplements off the menu, that would otherwise fill the nutrient gaps in our modern diets helping to prevent disease, it is only a matter of time until something in your body breaks, until something wears out, until something goes south, and then you have a health concern, you have a chronic disease, you've got blood pressure, you've got diabetes, you've got asthma, fibromyalgia, etc.

So you go to your doctor and he prescribes a drug for it. Let's say you've been diagnosed with asthma; well from my nutritional understanding, asthma has its root cause in nutrient deficiency, primarily a deficiency of essential fatty acids. You don't have asthma or for that matter any other chronic disease because you have "bad" genes. You don't get a chronic disease because you have a voodoo curse. You have a chronic disease because you have been given the wrong diagnosis! Your body has simply run out of the nutrients necessary to maintain and regulate its health, it's that simple!

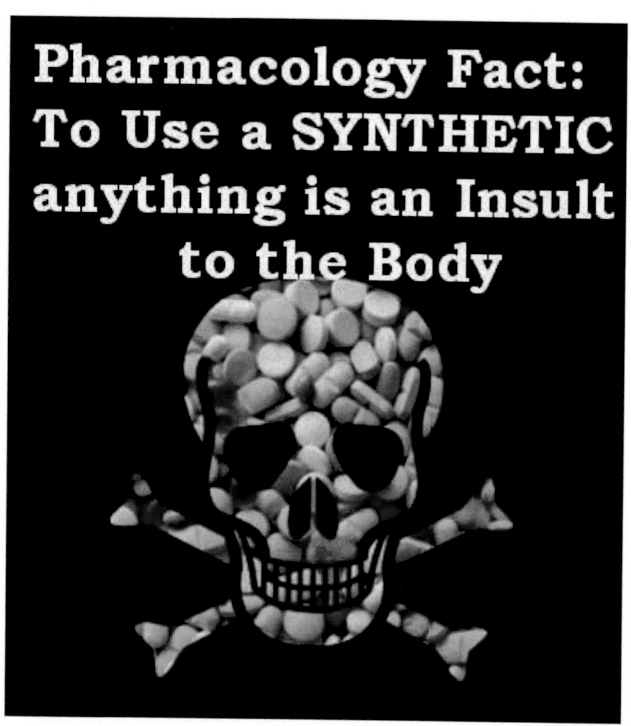

No drug actually reverses any disease. They merely mask symptoms while allowing the underlying causes of disease to worsen. Orthodox medicine has been monopolised by the pharmaceutical industry and as such, doctors receive no training in nutrition and so have no real understanding and certainly no clinical experience with nutrition. Medical doctors main focus is by and large, in the use of pharmaceuticals and surgery.

According to their medical paradigm once you get sick you are doomed! Your body cannot fix itself; it's the doctor's job to manage things with drugs until they get so bad that for example, if you suffer from arthritis, you will eventually have to seek a new hip or knee replacement and then five years later when that hip or knee fails, do you get a refund? No! You get another hip or knee if you can afford it!

Now drugs and surgery are great if you have a burst appendix or have a bullet lodged in your arm, if you are unfortunate to be involved in a car accident, if you've got third degree burns, if you've allowed your body's nutritional tank to become so depleted over time that you end up needing kidney dialysis or a liver transplant, that's the real domain of your medical doctor; that's what they are excellent at. But where they are not making real progress is everything else, everything that you normally go to your doctor for. And that's because your doctor hasn't been trained in nutritional science and so, doesn't understand or appreciate the basic premise that most chronic diseases have their roots in nutrient deficiencies.

Did you know that there are over 270 illnesses that can be caused by a calcium deficiency? High blood pressure is one of them; bad menstrual cramps are often caused by a calcium deficiency. An inability to fall asleep at night is a calcium deficiency most of the time. Muscle tics and cramps have their roots in calcium deficiency. Tinnitus (ringing in the ears) has its roots in a calcium deficiency. So you don't have a bad gene or a voodoo curse; most of the time you simply have a nutritional deficiency!

If you don't believe me, then take a look at the hordes of patients standing in line at the pharmacy. Do they look the picture of health? Most of them are most likely on multiple medications and they got there through their own fault. They most likely consumed excessive amounts of bad fats, too much sugar and too many over-processed foods, all of which contain few of the vitamins, minerals and essential fats their bodies needed to maintain health. Not to mention the "nutrient robbers" they frequently subjected their bodies to, such as excess alcohol, smoking, medications and stressful lifestyles. It's a very easy recipe for ill health!

If you want to have a healthy mind and body, feel alive and full of energy, then perhaps it's time to do what the healthy people do. I guarantee you that healthy people are consuming a diet of unprocessed whole foods, including plenty of fruits and vegetables, nuts and seeds, grains and other plant foods together with moderate amounts of fish, organic chicken and lean meats as well as some eggs and dairy products. All this in conjunction with: an active lifestyle, a positive mental attitude, and avoidance of smoking, excess alcohol and negative stress. These healthy individuals also take high quality nutritional supplements to help fill any nutritional voids that may otherwise occur in their diets from time to time.

Your Supplement Regimen

So the bottom line is that since food in the main is no longer very nutritional, your only recourse to maintaining good health is to supplement your diet with a selection of high-quality natural micro-nutrients. Remember though, the purpose of a nutritional supplement is to augment, not replace a healthy diet. Supplements can help in the prevention of illnesses resulting from inadequate nutrient intake, but will not substitute for a good diet.

The crucial question to consider then is: how much supplementation do we need? One thing is for sure, our bodies need far more that the Recommended Dietary Allowance suggests, as Dr. Cheraskin and as his SONA results show.(47) As there is no such thing as a well-balanced diet anymore, consequently the average so-called 'healthy' person is far from healthy. Especially when you consider the definition of health as proposed by the World Health Organisation, which states that: *"Health is not merely the absence of disease, it's a vibrant state of wellbeing and enjoyment of life".* Most so-called healthy people have low-energy levels, aches and pains, headaches, excess body weight, digestive issues, blood pressure problems, and difficulty sleeping!

When embarking upon a supplementation regimen, we must think about nutrient needs based on our individual requirements for optimum health. Luckily, for the most part, you don't have to go overboard with the amount of supplements you take every day. Just keep in mind that since nutrients work synergistically together, you should be taking a comprehensive regimen of daily vitamins, minerals, essential fatty acids and other nutrients as individually required.

So for a strong nutritional foundation, I recommend five key supplements you should be taking on a daily basis:

- Multivitamin/mineral complex
- Calcium/Magnesium with vitamins D3 and K2
- Coenzyme Q10 (CoQ10)

- Omega-3 fatty acids
- Probiotics

Multivitamin/mineral Complex

Think of these as your nutritional safety net. They fill the nutrient gaps in your diet helping to offset problems associated with poor dietary choices.

Calcium/Magnesium/Vitamins D3 & K2 Complex

Take these extra minerals and vitamins even if you already take a good multi-complex. You can take it as fact that you don't get enough of these nutrients in your daily diet. Researchers estimate that up to 80% of the population in the northern hemisphere are at risk of vitamin D deficiency. Vitamin D is necessary for the absorption and utilisation of calcium as well as for a healthy immune system. When supplementing with Vitamin D, it is also important to supplement with vitamin K2. Vitamin K2 works in conjunction with vitamin D to help move calcium into the proper areas in your body, such as your bones and teeth. These vitamins also help remove calcium deposits from areas in your body where it shouldn't be, such as your artery walls and soft tissues. So together they strengthen your bones while also improving cardiovascular health. Without adequate vitamin K2 levels within the body, prolonged intake of excessive doses of vitamin D may produce toxic effects, hence the need for supplemental K2 when taking vitamin D supplements.

Coenzyme Q10 (Co Q10)

Your cells need a constant supply of high-octane energy (ATP) to keep you in vibrant health. Co Q10 is the nutrient responsible for providing that initial energy spark to all 50 trillion cells in your body. This amazing molecule discovered back in 1957, plays a major part in producing over 95% of your body's energy requirements. When you're young, your liver produces CoQ10 in sufficient amounts to support bodily functions. However, as you age, your body's natural production of CoQ10 significantly decreases, which is why supplementation becomes so important. In addition, if you take cholesterol-lowering drugs called statins, your body's CoQ10 levels will decrease even further. Researchers found that these drugs deplete the CoQ10 in your body by as much as 50%. With insufficient levels of CoQ10 in your body, your cellular energy will decrease, and over time, can lead to some serious health problems including loss of vision, heart disease and dementia. To prevent a CoQ10 deficiency aim for 100mg – 200mg of CoQ10 (as ubiquinol) per day.

Omega-3 Fatty Acids

Omega-3 fatty acids form the building blocks of a number of anti-inflammatory compounds in our bodies with health benefits that are seemingly endless. Numerous studies have demonstrated that omega-3 fats protect the heart and help prevent heart attacks by making blood less likely to clot, increases good cholesterol while lowering the bad cholesterol and quells inflammation. Omega-3s also protect the brain from diseases like Alzheimer's, the eyes from developing cataracts, the joints from arthritis, along with a host of other health benefits too numerous to list here.

However, with our modern diets we consume an overwhelming amount of omega-6 fatty acids in proportion to omega-3 fatty acids. The diet of today contains a lot of salad dressings and processed foods made with vegetable oils, and these provide an overabundance of omega-6 fatty acids that literally promote inflammation inside your body, which ultimately leads to chronic health issues as you age.

To help balance the ratios of omega-3s to omega-6s, you must consume more cold-water fish such as salmon, herring, sardines, tuna, trout and mackerel. In addition, I recommend you take a daily omega-3 fish oil or krill oil supplement to make sure you get enough of this important nutrient.

Probiotics

In order to absorb the nutrients you are taking, it's imperative to have a healthy gastrointestinal tract, otherwise you won't get the full benefits of supplementation. This is where probiotics can help by boosting the friendly bacteria in our gut.

In the gut, beneficial bacteria are a naturally occurring phenomenon provided your diet is high in fibre and unprocessed foods, including naturally fermented foods like yoghurts and sauerkraut. Over 400 species of bacteria live naturally inside our digestive system. Most of these bacteria are beneficial to our health, aiding digestion, helping to nourish the cells lining the gut wall, producing important vitamins and supporting the immune system.

An imbalance of gut flora in your digestive tract (known as dysbiosis) can occur when the bad strains of bacteria get out of control causing inflammation and mal-absorption. Taking a high-quality probiotic every day ensures the beneficial bacteria in your gut always have the competitive edge.

The above nutrient recommendations serve as a basic regimen for establishing optimum levels of the micro-nutrients needed for good health. On the other hand, if we are trying to treat a particular health condition, then one must take into consideration the specific needs of the individual in question, as suggested by their particular condition along with their biological individuality, regarding sex, age, weight, activity levels and lifestyle choices. This is the point where consultation with a nutritional or naturopathic therapist would be helpful, because we are now entering an area where we are using nutritional supplements as therapeutic agents to treat disease.

High Quality and Natural – The Key

A word of advice when purchasing supplements; don't go cheap. Invest in high-end quality supplements based mostly on food concentrates. Nutrients derived from real foods are far healthier that man-made synthetic nutrients. It's important to know that not all natural supplements are created equal. Cheaper retail products made for the mass market may have ingredients whose quality and strength have been compromised. For instance, the manufacturing process may be speeded up, which can destroy some ingredients through excessive heat and compaction.

Also, low-cost products often contain reactive fillers and binders, which further reduce the expense of manufacturing. Reactive fillers commonly used to reduce expense and bulk-up the product include talcum powder, shellac, hydrogenated oils, gluten, yeast and lactose. Unfortunately, these fillers reduce both the biological activity and clinical effectiveness of the nutrients.

Additionally, how the nutrient is bound will also make a difference for ease of absorption and utilization. For example, iron sulphate is a commonly used form of iron that irritates the intestines and may cause constipation. The source of the problem here is not the iron but the sulphate carrier. Other forms of iron such as iron glycinate are less likely to cause constipation. A rule of thumb, when taking minerals, is to take them as either: citrates, fumarates, glucanates, amino acid chelates or picolinates.

To identify if a nutrient is synthetic, check on the label to see if a source is given. If it isn't, assume the product is synthetic. Terms that can identify a vitamin as synthetic include: hydrochloride, chloride, acetate, bitartrate, nitrate and succinate. In the naturally occurring forms of vitamins, for example: vitamin C complex, the ascorbic acid portion comprises only about 5% of the whole complex. Similarly, alpha-tocopherol only comprises a small percentage of vitamin E complex.

We as consumers have been thoroughly fooled and misled about vitamins and minerals. We have been hoodwinked into believing that large quantities of dead synthetic chemicals are more nutritionally potent than smaller amounts of high-quality natural living compounds. Relatively small amounts of whole-food natural nutrients with all of their naturally occurring synergists are far more potent than high doses of synthetic imitation vitamins and metallic-based minerals.

It is a natural law that you can't repair and rebuild a living body with dead synthetic chemicals. It simply isn't possible.

CHAPTER 10

THE PSYCHOLOGICAL AND SPIRITUAL SIDE OF HEALING

> *"Of one thing I am certain; the body is not the measure of healing Peace is the measure" – Phyllis McGinley*

In the early 1930s Dr. Edward Bach, an English physician wrote: *"Behind all disease lie our fears, our anxieties, our greed and our likes and dislikes"*.(48) He made this revolutionary statement upon personal observation of his many patients, whose physical ailments seemed to be predisposed by negative psychological or emotional states such as fear, anxiety, worries, jealousy, poor self-image, anger and resentment. He believed that for true healing to occur, these negative emotional states must be resolved. *"Treat people for their emotional unhappiness, allow them to be happy and they will become well"* he states.

In fact, Dr Bach's revolutionary ideas are not entirely new; all the great religions and philosophies abound with references to the effect the mind has on the body. The Bible says *"that as a man thinketh, so is he".(49)* Jesus, when asked about what food to eat said *"it is not what goes into the mouth that defiles someone but what comes out".(50)*

The old adage that "a healthy mind is a healthy body" is especially relevant in today's fast-paced society. If you are going to look at health purely from the nutritional side, you are going to miss living. You have to realize that it isn't just nutrition that gives zest and vitality to our lives. As well as feeding our bodies, we must also nourish our mind and soul.

Health, as I previously explained: is *'the attainment and maintenance of the highest state of mental and physical vigour of which any individual is capable'*. To this end, true health implies having vivacity and an appetite for life in all its aspects; of physical activity, of music and the arts, of fun and laughter, of fine conversation and philosophy, of friendship and of the capacity to love.

Although ill health is usually the culmination of a number of factors; things such as fear, insecurity, anxiety, frustration or anger can also bring on sickness. Most people don't realize that the mental faculties trigger the release of certain glandular secretions in the body. The mechanisms behind these secretions represent the connection between the mind and the body and these mechanisms have received intense scrutiny from medical researchers over the past thirty-plus years. This has led to a new field in medicine called psycho-neuro-immunology where studies have confirmed that the emotional and psychological state of a person influences a myriad of bodily processes for better or for worse.

How Emotions Harm *YOU.*

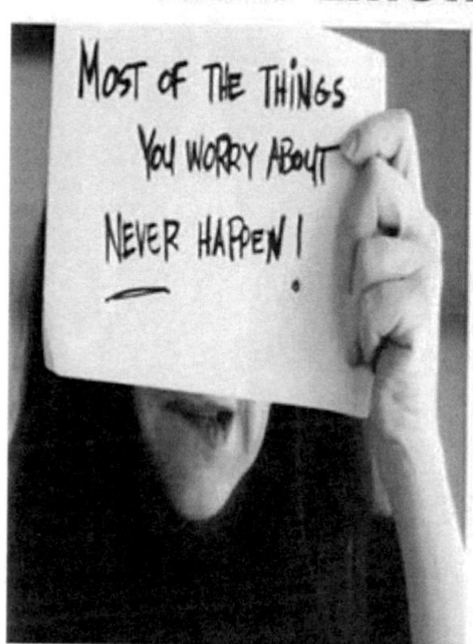

- **Anger** : ***Weakens The Liver***
- **Grief**: ***Weakens The Lung***
- **Worry** : ***Weakens The Stomach***
- **Stress** : ***Weakens The Heart & Brain***
- **Fear** :***Weakens The Kidney***

For example, our bodies have special in-built mechanisms to deal with stress, whether physical or psychological in origin. When our body perceives stress, our adrenal glands go into action and release the hormones adrenaline and cortisol. Both these hormones have a wide range of effects including increasing the heartbeat, reducing digestive activity in order to move blood away from these organs in favour of the muscles, heart and brain for fast action, and for releasing sugar and fats into the blood for fast energy. All this is very useful to escape imminent physical danger as in the classic "fight or flight" response.

But the positive side of stress only goes so far. Escaping an immediate danger as in a predator, for example, only takes seconds or minutes, and once the immediate danger is over the system is returned to a state of relaxation. However, if one is overwhelmed by constant psychological stress, never getting a break for months or years, then the stress never gets resolved and so the body never returns to its normal state of relaxation. Our bodies were never designed for this type of scenario!

Like the constant dripping of water, the accumulated effects of negative psychological states such as anger, fear, resentment and anxiety will gradually exhaust the adrenal glands leading to burn-out. This continuous physiological arousal of the adrenals can take its toll, eventually leading to chronic fatigue, poor immunity and ongoing low-grade inflammation that leads to a host of chronic diseases including diabetes, obesity and heart disease.

Our bodies work differently when under physical or psychological stress. That's why we're more prone to suffer from muscular tension, poor digestion and increased blood pressure as a result of prolonged stress. The effect of stress reduces the body's ability to absorb nutrients from the diet, including calcium, vitamin C,

Stress-Induced Health Problems

Stress can influence endocrine function, the immune system and the brain. The following conditions are commonly linked to stress:

- Angina
- Asthma
- Auto-immune diseases
- Cancer
- Depression
- Diabetes (Type 2 adult onset)
- Headaches
- Hypertension
- Immune suppression
- Irritable bowel syndrome
- Menstrual problems
- Ulcerative colitis
- Ulcers (gastric & duodenal)

Source: Selye, H. Stress in Health and Disease (Butterworths, 1976)

and numerous others. Also, when under stress, the body excretes more magnesium and potassium via the kidneys. Because calcium, magnesium and potassium are important for the proper regulation of muscular tension, their depletion explains why stress can cause muscular spasms and cramps. So, when we suffer from mental tension it produces physical tension where all the muscle structures of the body wear out more quickly: the cells of a tight muscle deteriorate more quickly and so has to be repaired more often.

The body is the servant of the mind. It obeys the operations of the mind whether its thoughts are deliberately chosen or automatically expressed. It is a truism that many diseases are started in the mind and conversely many diseases are relieved by a change of mental and emotional thinking.

When we are suffering from ill health we need to also look in other directions besides the physical. There are attitudes with our jobs, with our families and with the ups and downs of life. These attitudes can either build or destroy. It's ironic that one of the few things in life over which we have full control is our attitudes towards what life throws at us and yet most of us live our entire lives believing we have no control whatsoever. It is our attitudes that determine our physical health. Those who live in constant fear and worry of disease are the people who get it. If you are vindictive or malicious you produce tension in your body. When you feel hurt and rejected, there is tension in the body. When emotions such as hate or fear develop, they begin in the head first and then slowly seep into the body like poisons. To give someone a piece of your mind, you have to give up peace-of-mind!

Most of us blame people, situations and things "out there", for making us angry, sad, or distressed. Yet it is not the outside things that cause us stress, but our inside perceptions that cause our emotional turmoil. Understanding your emotions allows you greater control over negative feeling like anger and anxiety.

Emotions such as fear, hate or anger can cause congestion, resulting in blood pooling in some part of the body. Fear can bring on a balanced face. Where does the blood go? If blood pools in a particular place of the body for a period of time, blood clots may form and result in strokes or even a heart attack. Negative emotions like fear and anger are also known contributors to high blood pressure. Thoughts of malice, envy or sadness rob the body of its health and beauty. As a wise man once said: *"A sour face does not come by chance; it is the result of sour thoughts".(51)*

You must realise that you cannot starve you mind of positive thoughts and emotions and expect to have good health. Change of diet alone will not help the individual to greater health, who will not change their negative thought patterns. Sure, there are foods we can eat to improve for example: our digestion, but don't you think that your digestion can be affected by the way you think? For instance, the liver cannot function properly and the stomach cannot digest properly when these organs are bound up with worry and tension. To be honest, it's not so much the kind of food that goes into a person that determines health, but the kind of person the food goes into.....

So, if you want to achieve perfect health then guard your mind. It goes without saying that a healthy dietary regime will alter the pattern of, and reduce the incidence of many diseases, but attention to diet alone is never enough to create true health. You really don't need to worry about your body first. Focus on straightening out your mental direction by addressing any overly negative pessimistic thoughts. Of course, we all have done our share of negative thinking but let's get over that part of our lives; let's be finished with negative thinking. Never let negative feelings tell your thinking what to do. Feelings can be oftentimes misleading.

What a shock it must be to discover that negative thoughts and emotions can destroy the body! Since this is so, don't you think that you ought to turn away from negative thoughts? If you want to be happy then stop choosing to be miserable, it's that simple.

From now on, if you endeavour to live your life based on the axioms in the box below, then truly, you will have found the roadmap to optimal health and deep inner peace.

Today is a good time to start:-

- Today I will start with a smile and resolve to be agreeable. I will not criticize. I refuse to waste my valuable time.
- Today I refuse to spend time worrying about what might happen. I am going to spend my time making things happen.
- Today I will not imagine what I would do if things were different; they are not different. I will make success with what material I have.
- Today I am determined to do things I should do, and I firmly determine to stop doing the things I should not do.
- Today I will not indulge in self-pity. Instead I will strive to be cheerful. I will take the time to appreciate and value the good things in life.
- Today I will act towards other people as though this might be my last day on Earth. I will not wait for tomorrow: *"don't they know tomorrow never comes"* (New World in the Morning by Roger Whittaker).

According to the ancient saying: *"All roads lead to Rome"(52);* so too have I travelled far and wide in my quest to find *"my truth"* and embrace and live it wholeheartedly. In my search for meaning and to live a life of fulfilment, I came across many great intellects, whose writings have eloquently deciphered the way to living an inspirational life. One among them whose writings fits neatly into this narrative is the author Don Miguel Ruiz and his book: ***'The Four Agreements'*** that encapsulate an inspirational code for living.(53) In summary:

The Four Agreements – Don Miguel Ruiz's Code for Life

Agreement 1 – Be impeccable with your word. Speak with integrity. Say only what you mean. Avoid using the word to speak against yourself or to gossip about other. Use power of your word in the direction of truth and love.

Agreement 2 – Don't take anything personally. Nothing others do is because of you. What others say and do is a projection of their own reality, their own dream. When you are immune to the opinions and actions of others, you won't be a victim of needless suffering.

Agreement 3 – Don't make assumptions. Find the courage to ask questions and to express what you really want. Communicate with others as clearly as you can to avoid misunderstanding, sadness and drama. With just this one agreement, you can completely transform your life.

Agreement 4 – Always do your best. Your best is going to change from moment to moment; it will be different when you are healthy as opposed to sick. Under any circumstances, simply do your best and you will avoid self-judgement, self-abuse and regret.

The prose poem, "**Desiderata**"(54) written by American writer Max Ehrmann (1872 – 1945) starts with the line: *"Go placidly amid the noise and haste, and remember what peace there may be in silence"*. This brings to mind an effective technique for overcoming negative emotional states. The technique is to 'go within' in quietness, to be absolutely silent. When we practice silence, free of all activity, motion or disturbance, we access a stillness of mind that helps us to put all aspects of our lives into clearer perspective. There is no explanation quite as effective as silence. That is why disciplines such as regular meditation and floatation therapy are excellent tools to access this deeper realm, where truth and wisdom reside. When practiced diligently this technique will over time, transform your awareness to that level as exquisitely describe by the poet Walt Whitman (1819-1892) in **"Leaves of Grass"**(55):

Leaves of Grass

I exist as I am – that is enough

If no other in the world be aware, I sit content

And if each and all be aware I sit content.

One world is aware and by far the largest to me and that is myself,

And whether I come to my own today, or in ten thousand or ten million years;

I can cheerfully take it now, or with equal cheerfulness I can wait.

An Exercise in Self-Healing

Sit comfortable in a chair and close your eyes. Take three deep breaths, breathing in slowly to a count of five. Hold for a few seconds and then gently breathe out fully.

Then become aware of your whole body, starting with the top of your head. Allow the attention to pass over the whole body from the top of the head all the way down to the soles of the feet, and observing any tensions held in the body, let them go.

Repeat the word "relax" silently in your mind to help let go of any tensions that you become aware of.

In that awareness let the mind become free of any concern or preoccupation.

Each time other thoughts distract you, just let go of them and return to that inner awareness and come to rest within.

- Now be aware of your feet on the ground;
- The weight of your body on the chair;
- The texture of the clothes on your skin;
- And the play of air on your face and hands.
- Now, place your awareness on the senses:
- Be aware of smell……

- Be aware of taste……
- Be aware of hearing; of sounds near and far. Allow sounds to be received and let them rise and fall without comment or judgement of any kind……
- With your body completely relaxed and the mind clear, simply rest in this great awareness for a few minutes.

Symptoms of Inner Peace

Be on the lookout for symptoms of inner peace. The hearts of a great many have already been exposed to inner peace and it is possible that people everywhere could come down with it in epidemic proportions. This could pose a serious threat to what has, up to now, been a fairly stable condition of conflict in the world.

Some signs and symptoms of inner peace:

* A tendency to think and act spontaneously rather than on fears based on past experiences.

* An unmistakable ability to enjoy each moment.

* A loss of interest in judging other people.

* A loss of interest in judging self.

* A loss of interest in interpreting the actions of others.

* A loss of interest in conflict.

* A loss of the ability to worry. (This is a very serious symptom.)

* Frequent, overwhelming episodes of appreciation.

* Contented feelings of connectedness with others and nature.

* Frequent attacks of smiling.

* An increasing tendency to let things happen rather than make them happen.

* An increased susceptibility to the love extended by others as well as the uncontrollable urge to extend it.

WARNING:
If you have some or all of the above symptoms, please be advised that your condition of inner peace may be so far advanced as to not be curable. If you are exposed to anyone exhibiting any of these symptoms, remain exposed only at your own risk.

www.goyourownway.org

Page 1 of 1

CHAPTER 11

SPECIALIST DIAGNOSTIC TESTS

> *"There is only one health, but diseases are many. Likewise, there appears to be one fundamental force that heals; although the myriad schools of medicine all have their favourite ways of cajoling it into action" – Dr. Robert Becker*

In order to achieve a successful outcome for any health ailment, one first needs to get an accurate diagnosis of the underlying causes or conditions that are contributing to the illness. To this end whenever a client visits my health centre for treatment, as part of their assessment I employ a comprehensive range of specialist diagnostic tests such as Iridology, Live Blood Analysis, Magnetic Body Analysers, and subtle energy testing equipment including The Eductor and the Magnetspace 3D Non-Linear Diagnostic System, to help pinpoint the root causes of my client's health problems. Only then am I in a position to apply the best treatment strategies for a successful outcome as regards their health.

Following is a brief overview of each of the above mentioned diagnostic tests I use in my practice.

IRIDOLOGY: What your eyes reveal about your health

IMAGINE THIS: Someone you've never met looks in the coloured part of your eyes and gives you a detailed description of you, including your inherited strengths and weakness, your current health status in general, and the state of every organ in your body. Then, before you can recover from your astonishment, you realise that your eyes have somehow "video-taped" your entire life!

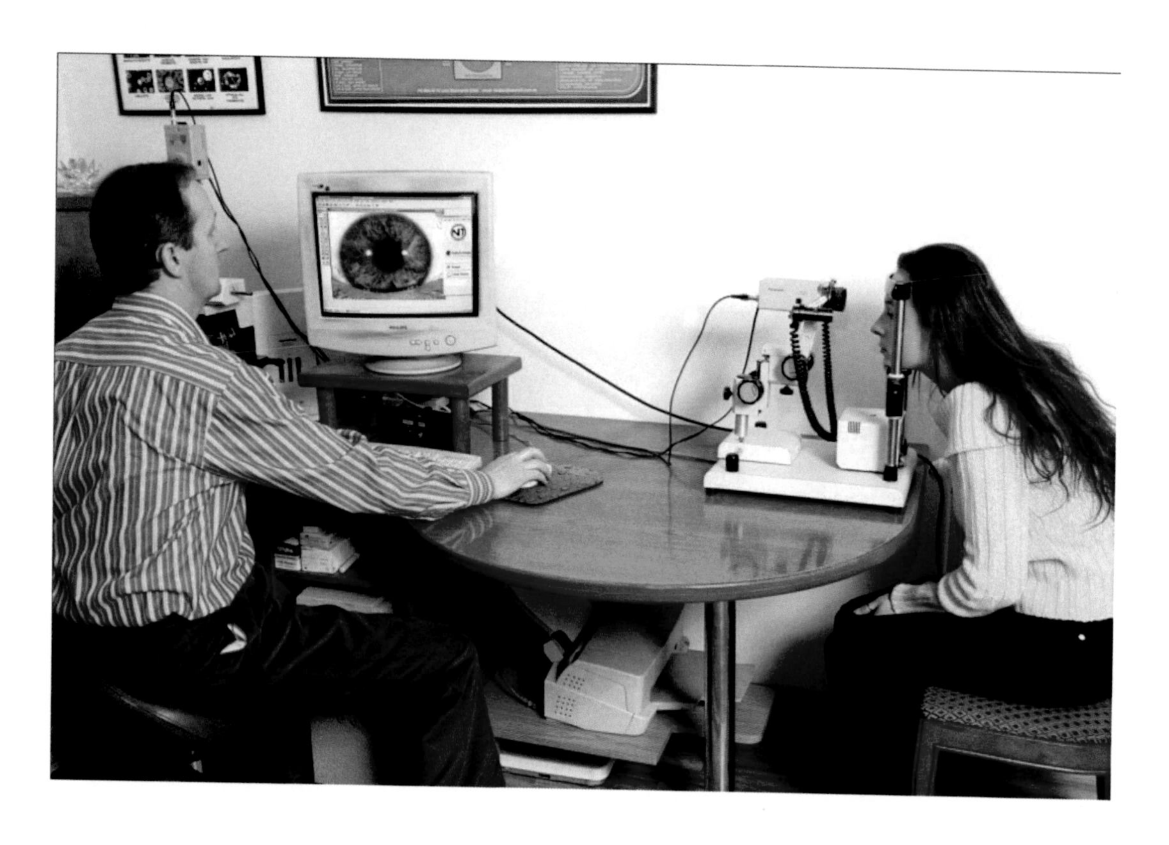

Proclaimed throughout the ages as the "window of the soul", the eyes also mirror changing conditions of every organ and tissue in the body.

Not just windows to the soul, your eyes reveal all: - health, physical weaknesses and even emotional attitudes. Through the structure of the iris nature has provided us with an invaluable insight into the health status of any individual through the science of iridology (pronounced: er-ri-dology).

Aside from the brain, the iris (coloured area encircling the pupil), is the most complex tissue structure of the whole body. Via a reflex mechanism, it is connected to every organ and tissue of the body by way of the brain and the nervous system and it works as a display unit of everything that takes place in our bodies.

With over 28,000 nerve endings located in each iris, these nerves fibres receive and register impulses from elsewhere in the body. These nerve fibres respond to both tissue and organ conditions with a corresponding physiological reflex that is manifested in the iris in the form of various markings, colour variations, and changes in texture or shape in the iris; all of which can indicate health concerns. Each eye gives us different information. The left eye correlates with the left side of our body and the right eye to the right side of our body.

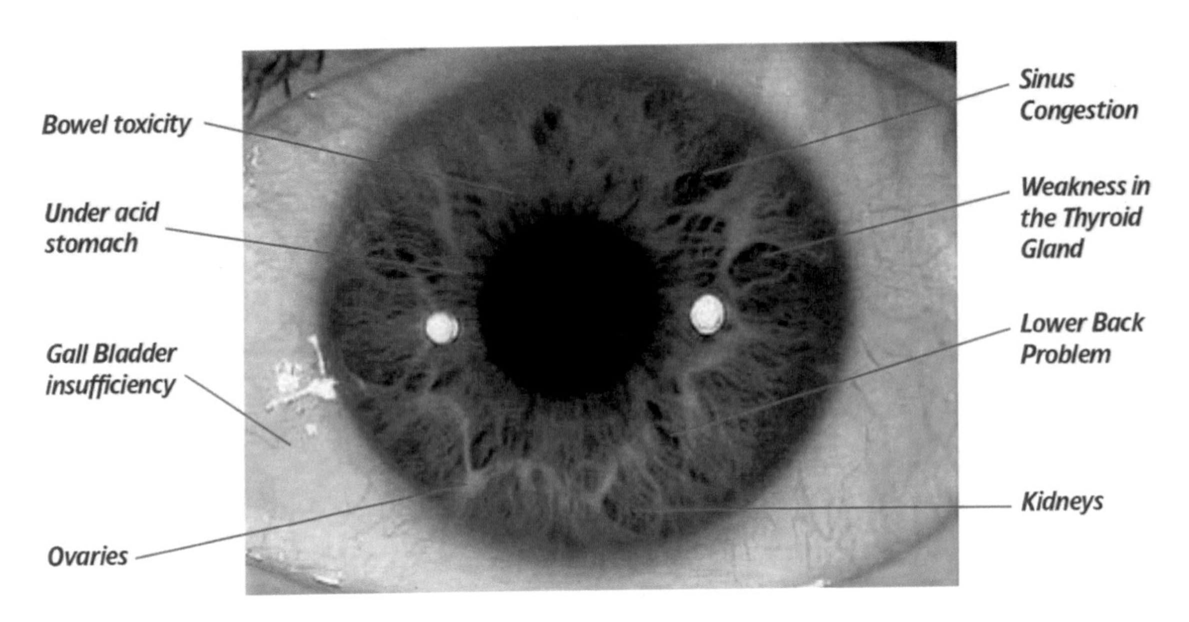

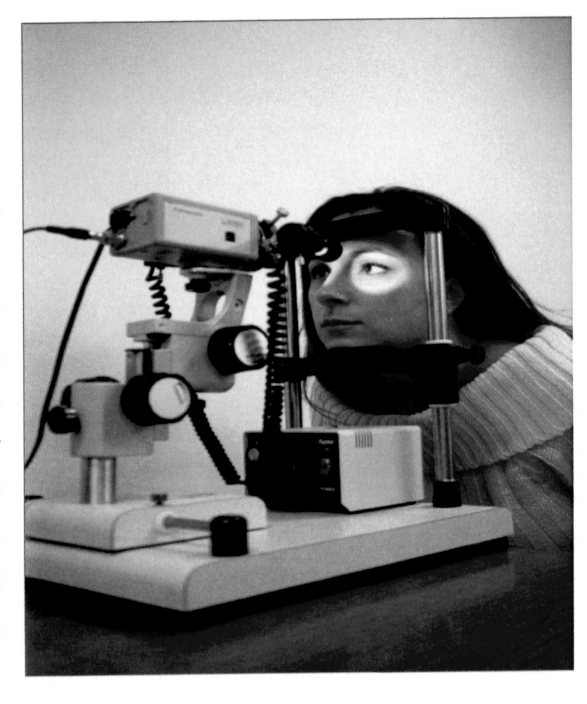

If you look closely at your iris, you may notice small dark spots, streaks or little openings in the fibres. These characteristics provide the key to understanding the state of health of each organ in your body. You can immediately gain insight as to whether your colon is inflamed, your thyroid is weak or underactive or your adrenals are over-stressed or burned out for example. You see the iris reflects the condition of the body tissues (e.g. inflammation, acidity, congested lymph, toxicity, hardened arteries, nerve weakness, etc).

The great advantage of iridology is that it lends itself handily to an immediate survey of the state of health of every part of a person's body. The iris will alert us to the early signs of approaching disease, and so appropriate preventative treatment can be taken to prevent subsequent illnesses that might otherwise follow.

I believe iridology to be a wonderful tool which helps confirm my diagnosis. It gives an overall "snapshot" of what makes up a patient. As clients enter my office they bring the diagnosis of their condition along with them, it is stamped in the iris of their eyes!

In this computer age, new technology has completely revolutionised the practice of iridology. We now have digital technology that allows us to see with great detail what the eyes have to tell us. At my clinic, I use a computer-assisted Digital Iriscope, which captures an image of the iris on a computer screen, and together with my client, I can discuss areas of concern.

Indeed, on many an occasion, I've had clients say to me during a session "how did you know that about me, we've only just met"? I remind them that: No I'm not psychic, but that their iris is like a fingerprint or a sort of blueprint of their genetic make-up and I'm able to read it like a map of their body to determine any risk factors to their health.

Also, our emotional and psychological states can be determined through various features in the iris. As emotional health and physical health go hand in hand, you will be given a "character reference" and we'll discuss how it may reflect on your health.

For instance, I can pinpoint the cause of health problems more effectively when I use iridology. Say for example a client comes to me suffering from migraine headaches, which may be caused by any number of reasons: - tension, hormonal imbalance, poor liver function, allergies or even spinal misalignment. By using iridology I can determine which area is the primary cause and so true curative and not just suppressant treatment can be given.

Recently, I had one case where a man who worked in construction was finding it difficult to work because of intense pain in his left foot, and no one seemed able to figure out why. When I studied his irises I found that the heel area of the left iris showed up as very white fibres indicating chronic inflammation. I put him on an alkalising diet and prescribed a course of anti-inflammatory herbs, which helped to dissolve what turned out to be a spur on his heel. He was fully cured within two months and no surgery was required.

Iridology reveals:	
1. The primary nutritional needs of the body 2. Constitutional strengths and weaknesses. 3. High risk tissue areas in the body that may lead to disease 4. Pre-clinical stages of potential diabetes, cardiovascular conditions and other diseases. 5. Depletion of minerals in any organ, gland or tissue. 6. A genetic pattern of inherent weaknesses and their influence on organs, glands and tissues. 7. Build-up of toxic material before the manifestation of disease.	8. Results of physical and mental fatigue or stress. 9. Source of infection. 10. The 'Whole' overall health level of the body as a unified structure. 11. Underactivity or sluggishness of the bowel. 12. Inflammation or ballooning of the bowel. 13. Nerve strength and nerve depletion. 14. Build-up of cholesterol and inorganic salts. 15. Lymphatic system congestion. 16. Poor absorption and assimilation of nutrients. 17. Personality traits and individual characteristics.

Iridology signs and their interpretation

Arcus Senilis

This is a classic sign associated with the onset of old age. It represents a lack of blood circulation to the brain. Symptoms such as headaches and vertigo may be experienced. Also, major brain functions may be declining such as memory and perception. People with dementia commonly have this sign.

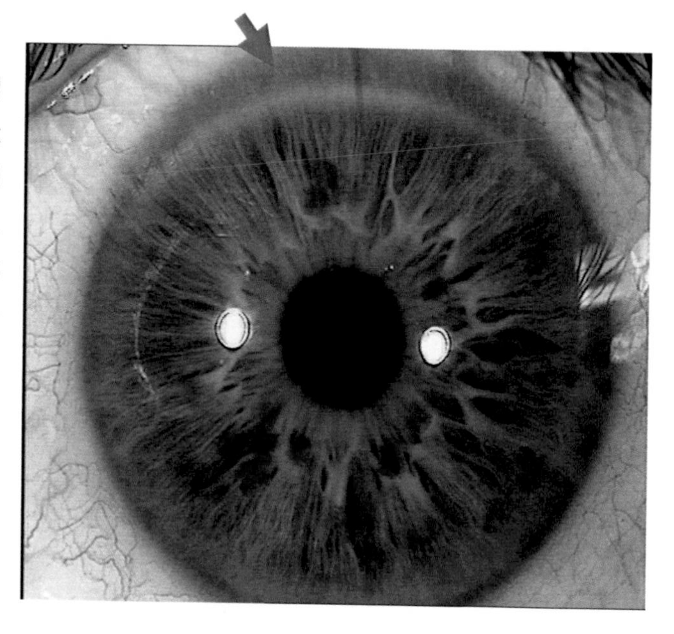

Lymphatic Rosary

Just inside the periphery of the iris are small white spots resembling a rosary beads. They indicate a predisposition to a congested or sluggish lymphatic system. The darker the spots the greater the toxic loading in the lymphatics. Symptoms can include lymphatic swelling from fluid retention, excess mucus and catarrhal production as in sinus problems and ear wax. Also women can experience tenderness and lumps in the breasts including cystic deposits anywhere in the body.

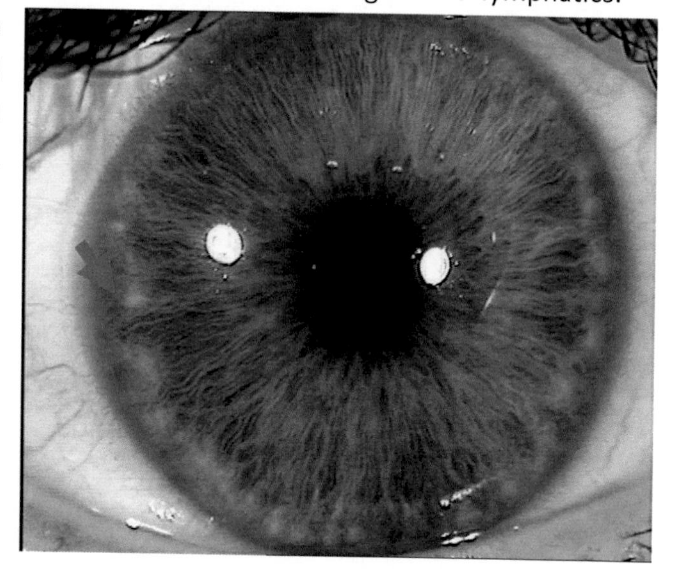

Nerve Rings

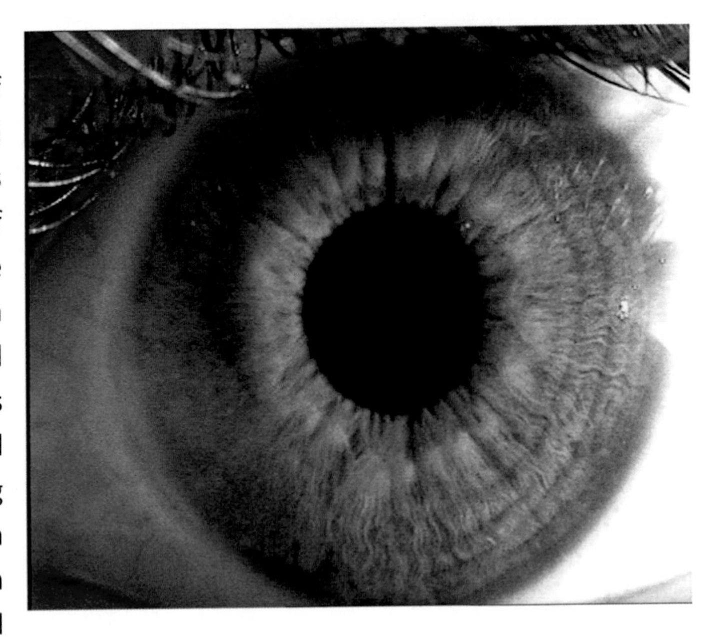

Observe a series of concentric rings spread throughout the iris. This indicates the degree of nervous tension in the individual as a result of both environmental and behavioural conditions. This affects the muscles and connective tissue, causing the muscles to stay in a contracted state, which results in stiffness and soreness as well as decreased circulation to various areas of the body. Nerve rings also indicate a degree of nervousness, anxiety and adrenal stress.

Ballooned Bowel

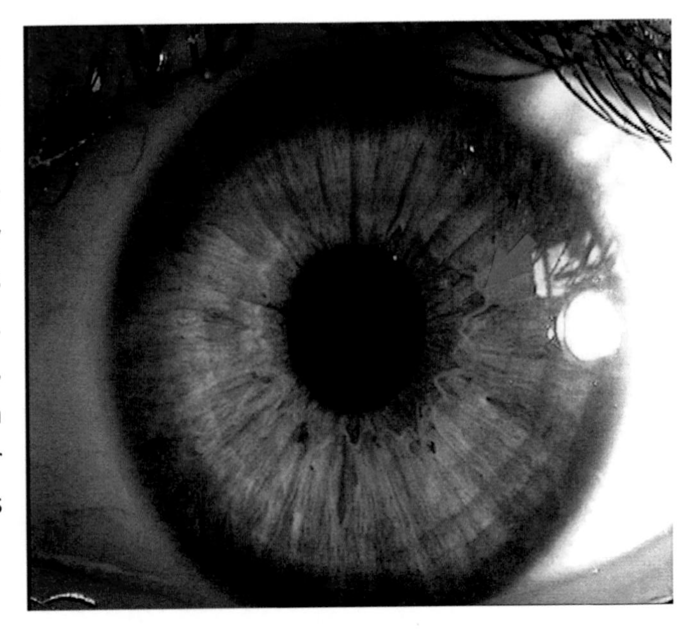

When the collarette is distended towards the periphery of the iris, this suggests a lack of tone in the intestines. Most commonly caused by constipation, gas and eating large meals. Symptoms include bloating, excess wind and sluggish bowels. The darker the colour in this area the more toxins located there.

Over acid Stomach

A bright white ring around the pupil indicates excess stomach acid production. Symptoms include belching, acid-reflux and heartburn.

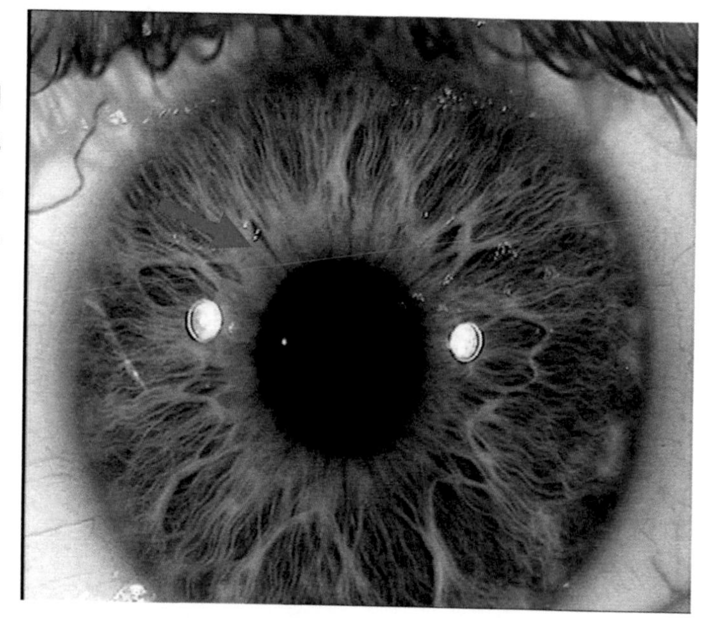

Radii Solaris

Observe dark spokes that radiate outwards like spokes in a wheel. They affect the organs or tissues through which the sign travels. These signs suggest altered circulation and lymph flow in these areas as a result of disturbed nerve trans-mission. They are also commonly associated with irritable bowel symptoms and depending on their locations can indicate psychological dispositions.

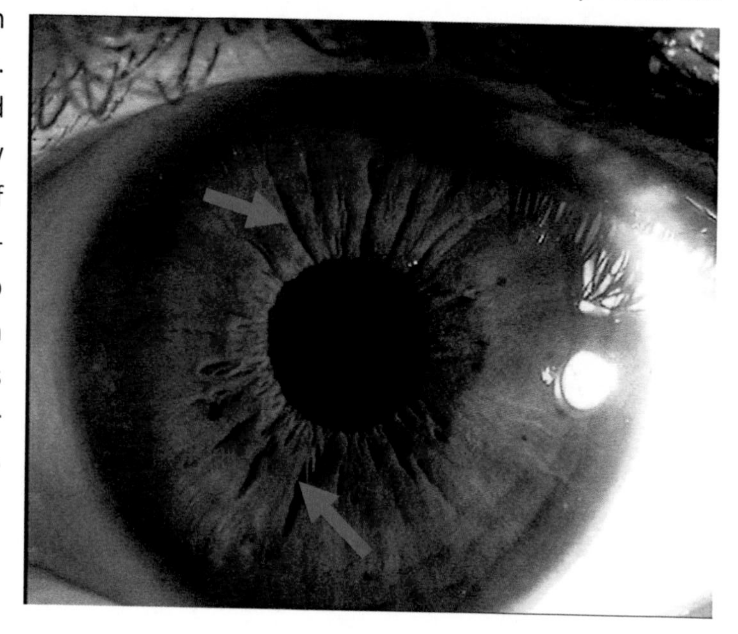

Live Blood Analysis

Live blood analysis (LBA) is a test that can give you a very accurate picture of your state of health and allows you to find out about any potential disease process occurring in your body.

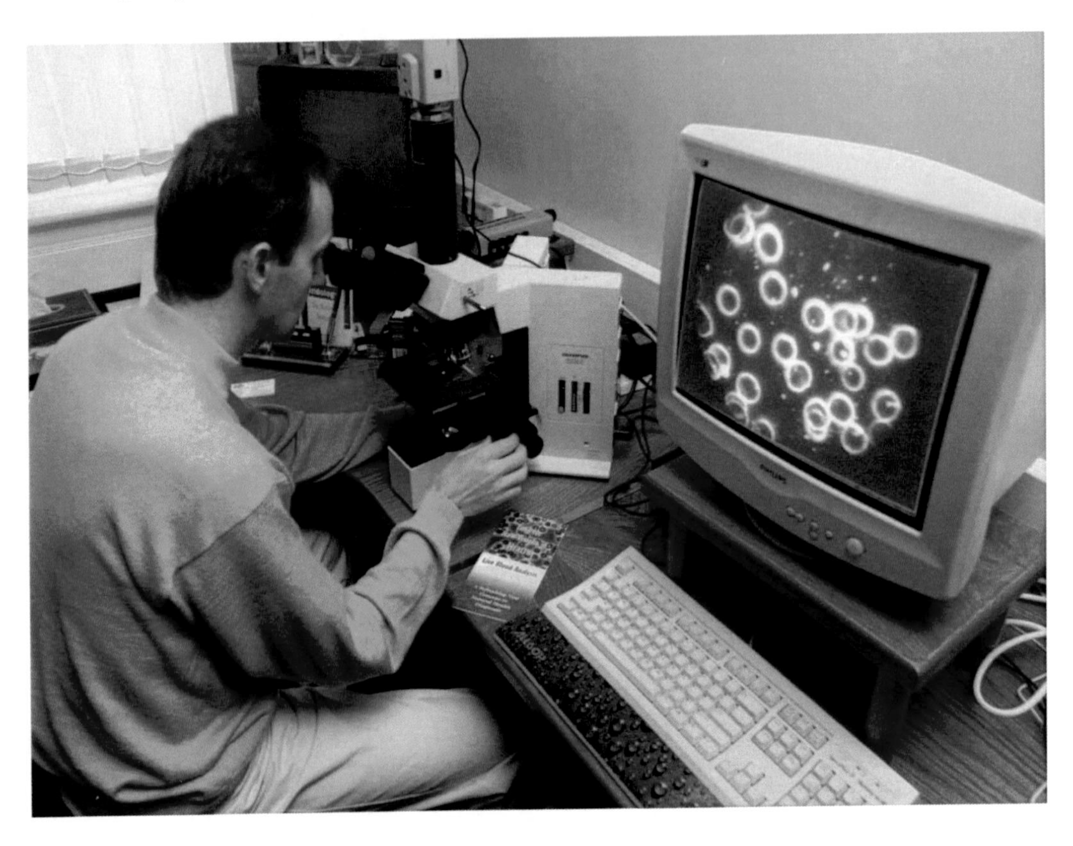

Also, known as **Darkfield microscopy**, it is the observation of live blood cells using a special microscope called a dark field microscope. Darkfield microscopy is a microscopic technique in which light strikes the sample being viewed from the side rather than from underneath. Therefore, the blood does not have to be dried or stained beforehand, and so the blood elements can be seen in their living state, hence the term "live blood" analysis.

How does it work?

The test is carried out by taking a drop of blood from your fingertip and magnifying it by 15,000 times. The blood is then shown on a video monitor and assessed while it remains active for up to twenty minutes. During the analysis you can see the contents of your own blood on the video screen where various states of sub-par health can be displayed through blood pictures that deviate from normal.

Seeing your own blood live on screen in front of you is fascinating and often profoundly moving. You can observe the shape and mobility of the red blood cells that deliver oxygen, watch the white blood cells as they devour toxins and invaders and observe the smaller platelets responsible for clotting. The state of the plasma fluid that these cells travel in is also discernible; and all from only a small drop of blood!

This blood picture you see gives fascinating clues about how well your body is dealing with life. Nutrition, water intake, environmental pollutants, toxicity and stress all affect the state of your blood which, as the delivery system to your cells, has a direct impact on many aspects of your health.

In a healthy individual, the blood is perfectly balanced with red blood cells that are uniform in shape and size (not elliptical, jagged or varying in size). Neither are the blood cells overlapping or clumped together but are loose and free flowing. The white blood cells although much fewer in number, are easily discernible due to their size (approximately twice as large as red blood cells) and also by their amoeba-like movements. The plasma is also clear and free of any fibrous material, platelet aggregation, or other artefacts.

Having such a close look at ourselves lets us see what is working well and what we might want to think about changing. Not only can the content and vitality of the blood be seen, but an immediate assessment can be made of a range of indicators of poor health.

Fat plaques in the blood, for example, are easily identifiable, as are the effects of fungal or pathogenic infections. Liver spicules that appear in the blood as long needle-like projections indicate liver stress or damage to liver cells. The presence of smaller than normal red blood cells indicates an iron deficient state and possible anaemia. Other borderline or chronic anaemia's due to vitamin B12 and folic acid deficiency can be depicted through the presence of larger than normal red blood cells. Red blood cells that are clumped together or excessive numbers of damaged and misshapen blood cells can grossly fatigue their owner due to their incapacity to deliver oxygen around the body.

The presence of different coloured crystals in the blood sample tells us even more. For example, yellow crystals indicate elevated serum uric acid concentration, common in people suffering from gout, poor kidney function, or are grossly dehydrated. Red crystals are indicative of bowel toxicity and also with liver toxicity. There are many other indicators we can observe in a live blood analysis that can pinpoint weaknesses in your body-organ systems that are not readily detectable through routine Blood Pathology tests.

Picking up on health problems in their early stages and even when symptoms are not yet specific, makes live blood analysis the ultimate preventative medical tool available today. Unlike normal Blood Pathology, these tests are performed in your presence allowing for on the spot feedback and interactive discussion over your treatment program. By being able to identify and treat health problems in their early stages is obviously beneficial to both the individual and their healthcare budget. Also, subsequent live blood screenings will show the client the benefits of the treatment they are receiving in their improving blood picture.

Is your blood a picture of health?

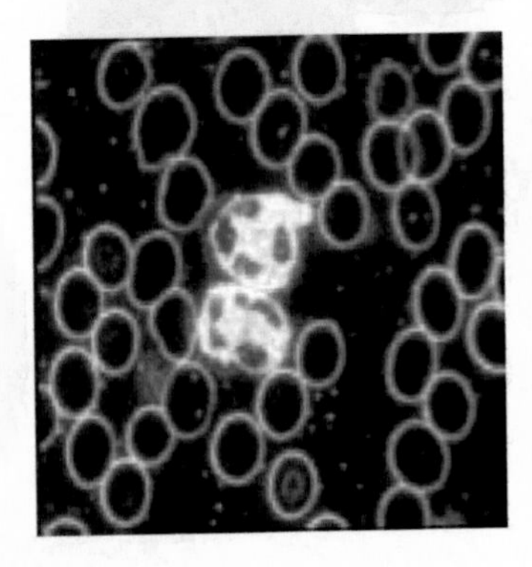

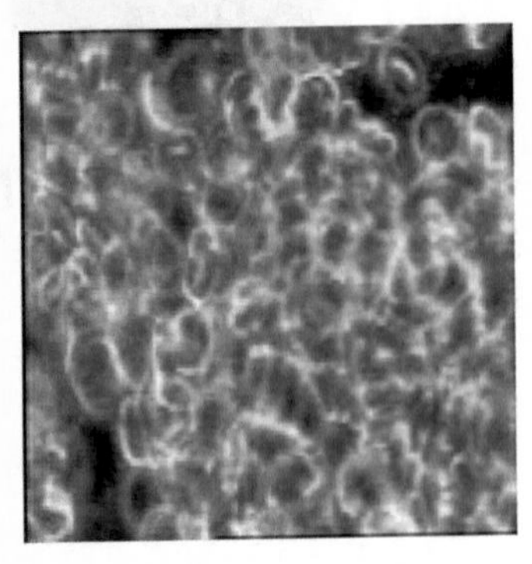

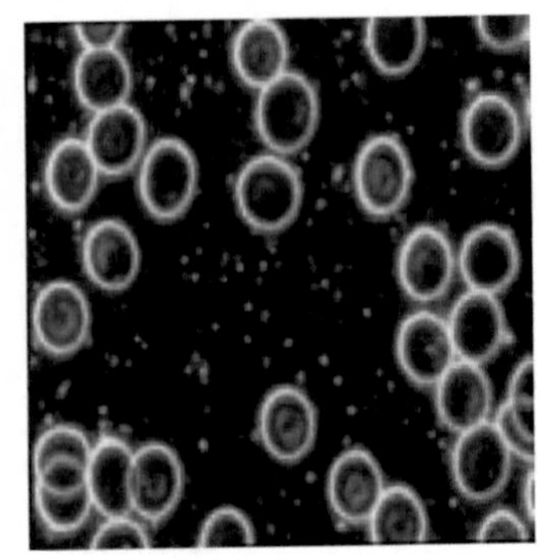

Information provided by Live Blood Analysis

Live blood analysis is a qualitative test to detect functional imbalance in the body including:

- Nutrient deficiencies (e.g. essential fatty acids, iron, vitamins, B9, B12, antioxidants and lipotropic (liver) nutrients).
- The immune system and how well it is functioning.
- pH imbalances (i.e. over-acidity)
- Digestive competence and gut permeability.
- Circulatory problems
- The condition of the liver
- Inflammation in the body.
- Presence of bacterial, parasitic or fungal forms.
- Detects numerous indicators of free radical stress and immune impairment, known precursors to chronic inflammation and disease pathology.

Case Study:

A 26 year old woman presented at my clinic suffering from recurring mouth ulcers, repeated respiratory tract infections and chronic fatigue. As a twelve year old girl she had been diagnosed by her doctor with pernicious anaemia, a condition caused by too little vitamin B-12 in the body. The treatment for pernicious anaemia is a series of vitamin B12 injections which she duly got.

However, since then, whenever she presented to her doctor suffering from fatigue and low immunity, they blamed her symptoms on low vitamin B-12 and suggested more vitamin B-12 injections. She duly complied. But this time she felt no better and over the years her symptoms just kept getting worse. She was referred to consultants who could find no other causes to explain her symptoms and again recommended more vitamin B-12 injections. So when she presented to my clinic I decided to do a live blood analysis to determine if she was indeed deficient in vitamin B-12. If she was, then I should see a number of macrocytes in her blood picture (excessively large red blood cells). The blood sample **(image 1)** showed no signs of macrocytes, but what I did observe were a very high number of poikilocytes and echinoytes (abnormally shaped red blood cells resembling a cogwheel). This crumpling of the membrane wall of the red blood cells is indicative of free radical damage. This damage may be due to various factors, or a combination of factors such as an essential fatty acid deficiency, antioxidant deficiencies (e.g. vitamins A, C & E), as well as exposure to heavy metals, infectious agents, allergies and a leaky gut.

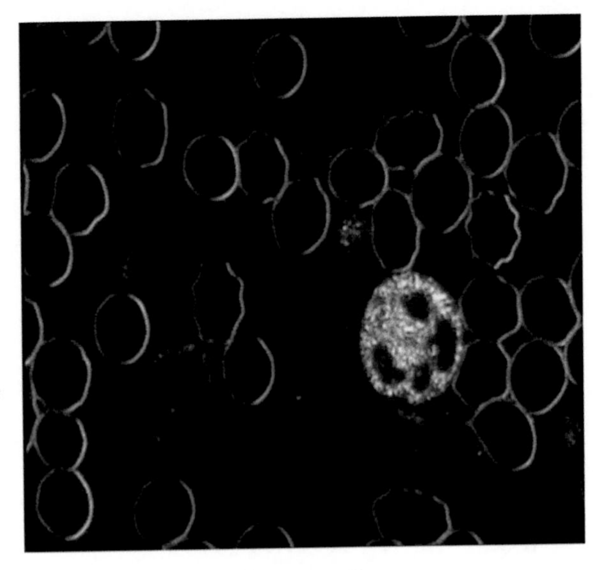

Image 1

Her treatment plan consisted of antioxidant nutrients to protect against oxidative damage to her red blood cells, omega-3 fatty acids with vitamin E which are both vital to the maintenance of cell membrane integrity; and also a combination of herbs to repair her leaky gut and support liver detoxification.

Image 2

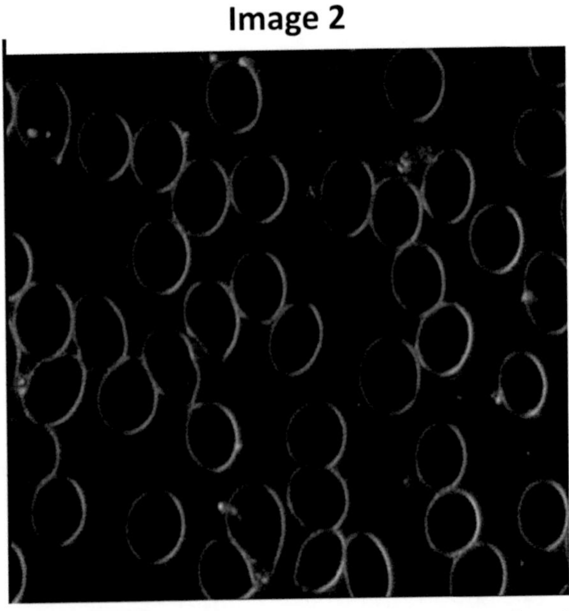

After three months on this protocol her energy levels returned to normal, mouth ulcers were gone and she suffered no more colds or flu. An analysis of her blood **(image2)** revealed a healthy blood picture with no jagged red blood cells evident; instead her blood cells were round and uniform in shape and size.

Various forms of Live Blood Images

Healthy Live Blood

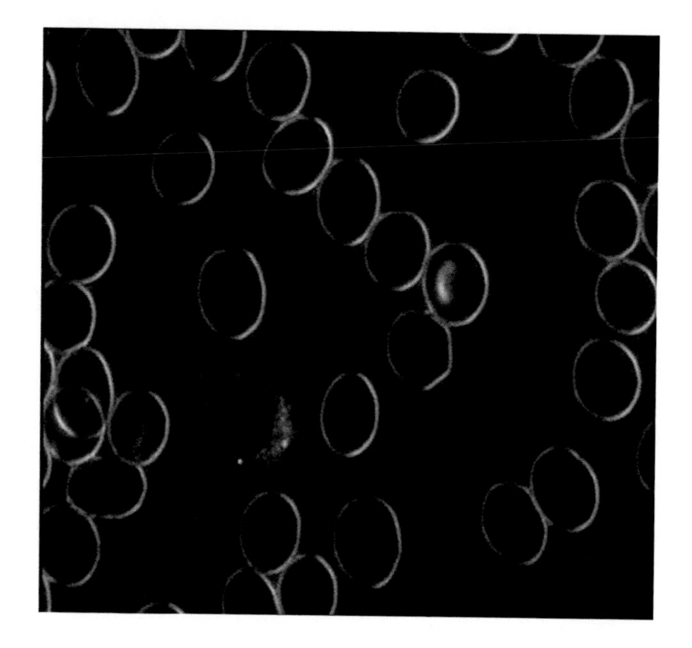

The cells are of even size and shape and are not sticking to each other.

Red Blood Cells in Rouleaux formation (stacking in long rows like a roll of coins)

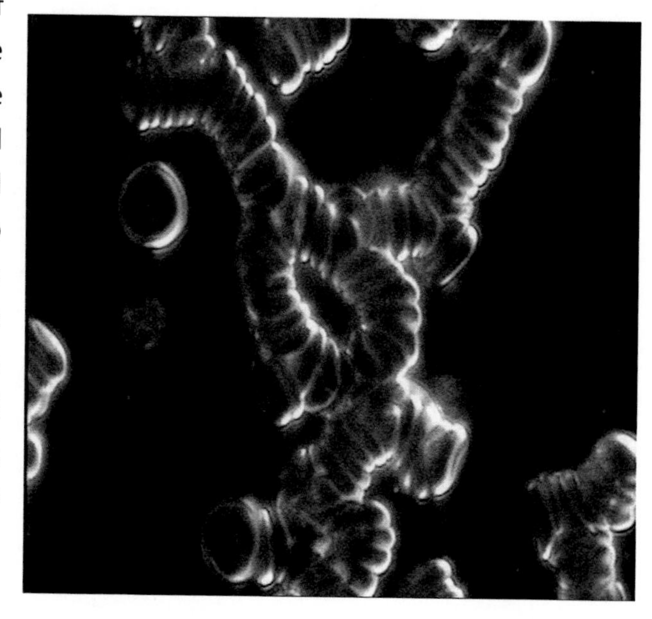

This is an indicator of inflammation equivalent to the erythrocyte sedimentation rate (ESR) of standard blood pathology. There is a decreased ability of the red blood cells to absorb and transport oxygen; hence fatigue is common with this picture. Such formations can be the result of dysfunctional digestion, food allergies, and underlying inflammatory processes.

High levels of fat in the blood (Chylomicrons)

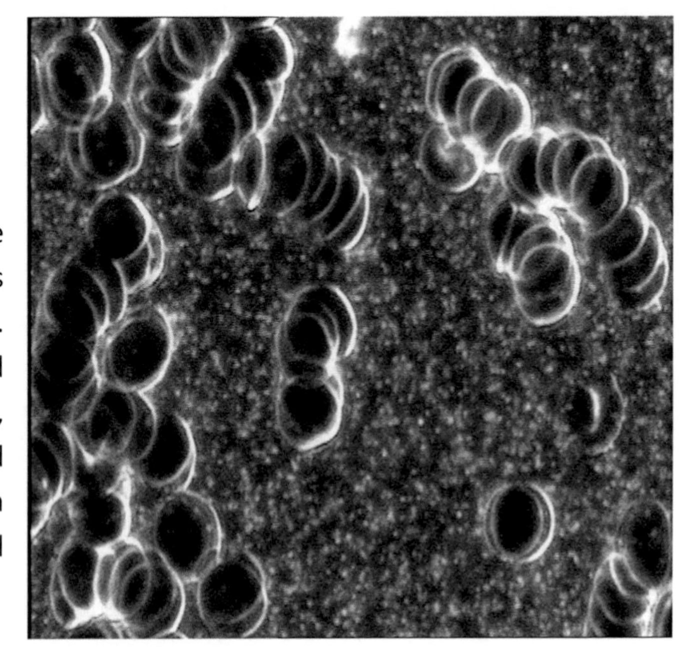

Observe the blood sample teeming with white flecks shimmering in the plasma. High fat levels in the blood promote heart disease, enlargement of the liver and poor tissue oxygenation, with resultant physical and mental fatigue.

Blood Picture showing two White Blood Cells (Neutrophils)

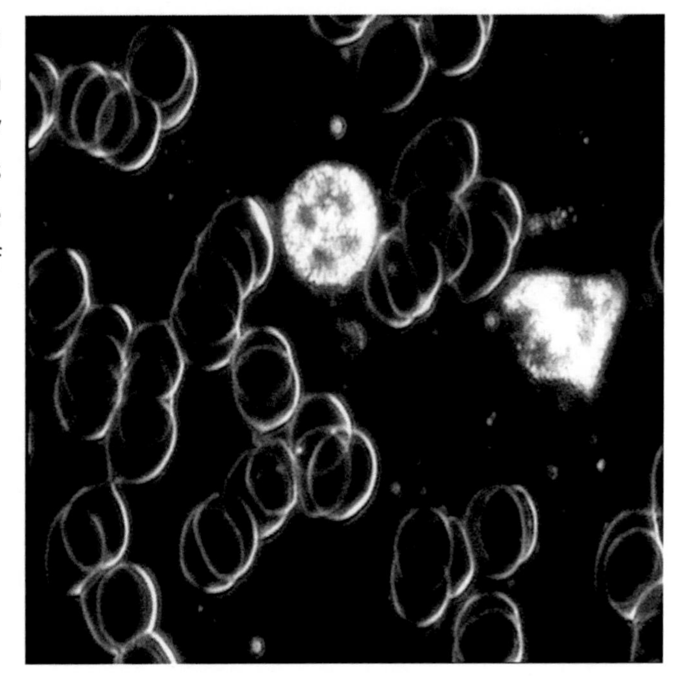

Live Blood Analysis can determine a lot about an individual's Immune status by observing both the quantities and degree of activity of the four different types of immune cells: -

- Lymphocytes
- Monocytes
- Neutrophils
- Eosinophils

Fibrin Spicules

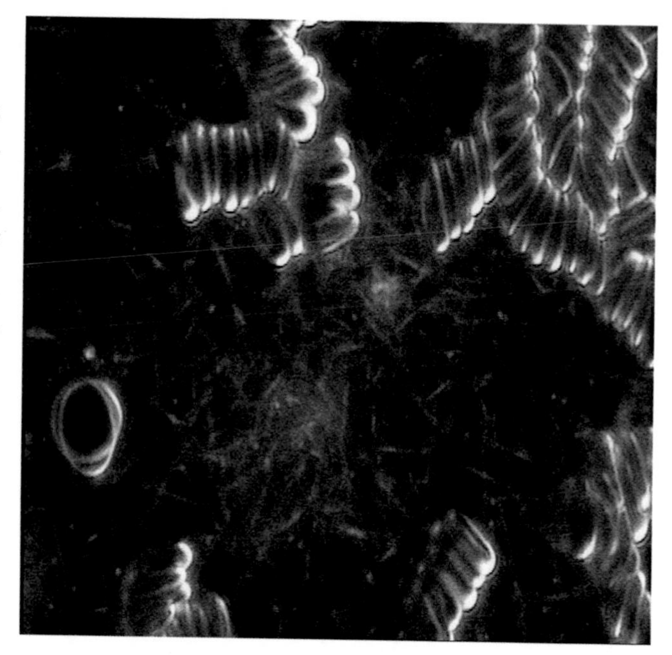

Clustered spike-like projections in the plasma, indicating liver dysfunction and/or damage. This may be a result of excessive use of drugs, alcohol, or a lifetime of poor dietary habits.

Thrombocyte Aggregate (Blood Clot)

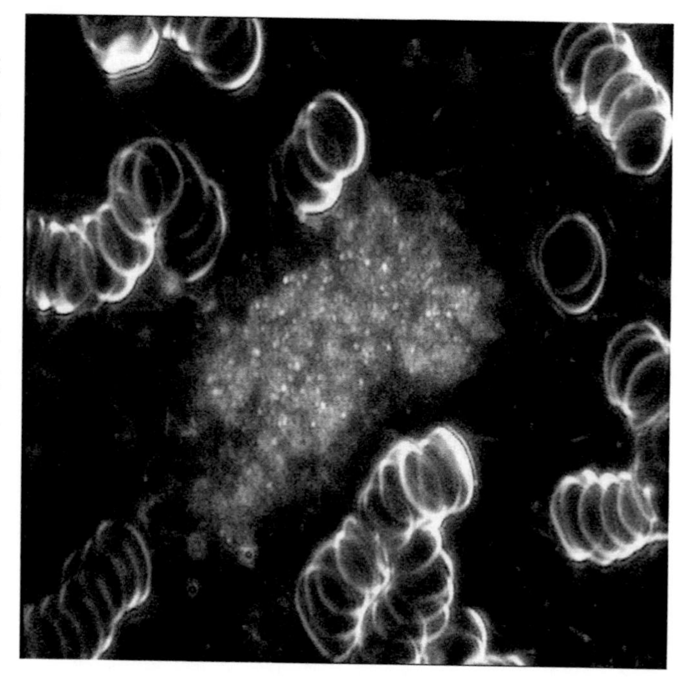

This is an indicator of platelet activation and poses a serious cardio-vascular risk. These aggregates can block small capillaries and impair circulation. In large amounts they may form clots, which can result in strokes or heart attacks. Blood clots may be due to smoking, high cholesterol, gut dysbiosis, chronic inflammation, stress or accelerated ageing.

Magnetic Human Body Analyser

"Electromagnetic energy is the primary form of energy on which every living organism depends"(56)

Electromagnetic energy and the human body have an important inter-relationship. The human body produces subtle magnetic fields that are generated by chemical reactions within the cells and also by weak electrical currents of the brain and nervous system. Our bodies function by way of these finely co-ordinated networks of electro-magnetic fields, which help regulate all bodily functions and keep them in their natural balance.

When the body's magnetic frequency patterns become disturbed, it is often the start of a chain of effects that leads to ill health. The body's first signal that all is not well is vibrational or electromagnetic in nature. These altered frequencies are stored in our cells and become damaging. They cause biochemical changes in cells affecting cellular function and ultimately leading to the development of pathologies.

To put it another way, when the magnetic frequency of our cells are high, we experience good health. When the frequencies of our cells are low, we are more susceptible to disease.

With the advent of Quantum Physics and from that Quantum medicine has evolved, scientists are now able to identify the specific electromagnetic frequencies of healthy body tissues and organs. When these frequency patterns deviate from their normal amplitude, it signifies stress in those tissues. These altered frequency patterns can now be detected long before any physical symptoms of disease appear. The more damage occurring in an organ or tissue, the more distorted the frequency patterns emanating from those diseased tissues become.

With this understanding medical engineers were able to build a device that can measure the electromagnetic energy emanating from the body's viscera. Any deviations in the frequency patterns outside of the normal range can be interpreted as a disease process occurring in those organs or tissues being tested.

The device I use in my clinic is called **"MagnetSpace"** and it has been calibrated to measure the different electromagnetic frequencies emanating from the human body. The system measures and analyse 27 different parameters relative to one's health status. They are:

Cardiovascular	**Vitamin/Minerals**	**Gastrointestinal**	**Gynaecology**
Liver Function	**Prostrate**	**Pancreas**	**Endocrine**
Blood Sugar	**Breast**	**Kidney**	**Immune System**
Lungs	**Amino Acids**	**Brain Function**	**Heavy Metals**
Bone Density	**Allergens**	**Rheumatic Bone**	**Eyes**
Adrenals	**Obesity Function**	**Toxins**	**Parasites**

With the MagnetSpace device I can identify many underlying pre-pathological conditions and diseases at their earliest pre-clinical stage when only some functional abnormalities are present, but not yet detectable by current medical tests. Following are some examples of the type of results obtained from this type of analysis:

Liver Function

Name: xxx xxxx Sex: Male Age: 44

Figure: Slightly heavier than the(172cm, 74kg) Testing Time: 2012-07-04 14:41

Actual Testing Results

Testing Item	Normal Range	Actual Measurement Value	Testing Result
Protein Metabolism	116.34 - 220.621	92.577	Mildly Abnormal (+)
Energy Production Function	0.713 - 0.992	0.669	Mildly Abnormal (+)
Detoxification Function	0.202 - 0.991	0.843	Normal (-)
Bile Secretion Function	0.432 - 0.826	0.684	Normal (-)
Liver Fat Content	0.097 - 0.419	0.503	Mildly Abnormal (+)

Cardiovascular and Cerebrovascular

Name: xxx xxxx Sex: Male Age: 44

Figure: Slightly heavier than the(172cm, 74kg) Testing Time: 2012-07-04 14:41

Actual Testing Results

Testing Item	Normal Range	Actual Value Measurement	Testing Result
Blood Viscosity	48.264 - 65.371	50.48	Normal (-)
Cholesterol Crystal	56.749 - 67.522	58.966	Normal (-)
Blood Fat	0.481 - 1.043	1.015	Normal (-)
Vascular Resistance	0.327 - 0.937	1.335	Mildly Abnormal (+)
Vascular Elasticity	1.672 - 1.978	1.747	Normal (-)
Myocardial Blood Demand	0.192 - 0.412	0.597	Moderately Abnormal (++)
Myocardial Blood Perfusion Volume	4.832 - 5.147	4.843	Normal (-)
Myocardial Oxygen Consumption	3.321 - 4.244	4.856	Mildly Abnormal (+)
Stroke Volume	1.338 - 1.672	1.551	Normal (-)
Left Ventricular Ejection Impedance	0.669 - 1.544	1.793	Mildly Abnormal (+)
Left Ventricular Effective Pump Power	1.554 - 1.988	1.601	Normal (-)
Coronary Artery Elasticity	1.553 - 2.187	1.864	Normal (-)
Coronary Perfusion Pressure	11.719 - 18.418	13.935	Normal (-)
Cerebral Blood Vessel Elasticity	0.708 - 1.942	1.691	Normal (-)
Brain Tissue Blood Supply Status	6.138 - 21.396	8.355	Normal (-)

Gynaecology

Name: xxx xxxx   Sex: Female   Age: 48

Figure: Standard body weight(166cm, 60kg)   Testing Time: 2012-07-05 18:24

Actual Testing Results

Testing Item	Normal Range	Actual measurement Value	Testing Result
Female Hormone	3.296 - 8.840	5.067	Normal (-)
Gonadotropin	4.886 - 8.931	2.186	Moderately Abnormal (++)
Prolactin	3.142 - 7.849	2.182	Mildly Abnormal (+)
Progesterone	6.818 - 16.743	9.75	Normal (-)
Vaginitis coefficient	2.204 - 2.819	2.742	Normal (-)
PID coefficient	1.348 - 3.529	5.258	Mildly Abnormal (+)
Appendagitis coefficient	2.301 - 4.782	2.755	Normal (-)
Cervicitis coefficient	2.845 - 4.017	3.984	Normal (-)
Ovarian cyst coefficient	2.012 - 4.892	7.866	Moderately Abnormal (++)

Bone Mineral Density

Name: xxx xxxx   Sex: Female   Age: 49

Figure: Slightly heavier than the(170cm, 70kg)   Testing Time: 2012-07-14 12:31

Actual Testing Results

Testing Item	Normal Range	Actual Measurement Value	Testing Result
Osteoclast Coefficient	86.73 - 180.97	88.947	Normal (-)
Amount of Calcium Loss	0.209 - 0.751	0.915	Moderately Abnormal (++)
Degree of Bone Hyperplasia	0.046 - 0.167	0.103	Normal (-)
Degree of Osteoporosis	0.124 - 0.453	0.469	Mildly Abnormal (+)
None Mineral Density	0.796 - 0.433	0.218	Mildly Abnormal (+)

Trace Elements and vitamins

Name: xxx xxxx Sex: Male Age: 44

Figure: Slightly heavier than the(172cm, 74kg) Testing Time: 2012-07-04 14:41

Actual Testing Results

Testing Item	Normal Range	Actual Measurement Value	Testing Result
Ca	61.431 - 78.329	59.436	Mildly Abnormal (+)
Fe	66.432 - 73.246	68.648	Normal (-)
Zn	1.143 - 1.989	1.67	Normal (-)
Se	0.847 - 2.045	1.866	Normal (-)
Pb	0.842 - 1.643	1.457	Normal (-)
Vitamin A	0.346 - 0.401	0.362	Normal (-)
Vitamin C	4.543 - 5.023	4.072	Mildly Abnormal (+)
Vitamin E	4.826 - 6.013	3.927	Moderately Abnormal (++)
Vitamin K	0.717 - 1.486	1.398	Normal (-)
Vitamin B1	2.124 - 4.192	2.274	Normal (-)
Vitamin B2	1.549 - 2.213	1.774	Normal (-)
Folic Acid	1.449 - 2.246	2.072	Normal (-)
Vitamin B3	14.477 - 21.348	16.694	Normal (-)
Vitamin B6	0.824 - 1.942	0.817	Mildly Abnormal (+)
Vitamin B12	6.428 - 21.396	8.644	Normal (-)
Vitamin D3	5.327 - 7.109	5.762	Normal (-)

Endocrine System

Name: xxx xxxx Sex: Male Age: 55

Figure: Severe partial fat(183cm, 95kg) Testing Time: 2013-05-03 14:20

Actual Testing Results

Testing Item	Normal Range	Actual Measurement Value	Testing Result
Thyroid secretion index	2.954 - 5.543	2.454	Mildly Abnormal (+)
Parathyroid hormone secretion index	2.845 - 4.017	2.528	Mildly Abnormal (+)
Adrenal glands Index	2.412 - 2.974	1.552	Moderately Abnormal (++)
Pituitary secretion index	2.163 - 7.34	0.772	Moderately Abnormal (++)
Pineal secretion index	3.210 - 6.854	2.442	Mildly Abnormal (+)
Thymus gland secretion index	2.967 - 3.528	3.255	Normal (-)
Gland secretion index	2.204 - 2.819	1.942	Mildly Abnormal (+)

ENERGY MEDICINE

We were all taught in secondary school science that we are made of atoms, and atoms are made of electrons, in spinning energy states, around protons and neutrons in the centre. Electrons don't ever touch because they are so charged. So no atom ever touches the next atom. And when I slap my hands together nothing touches anything, there is just repulsion of electrical fields. Instead, what we truly are, is an incredibly complex set of electro-magnetic-static-quantic and photonic fields!

According to Newtonian Physics all matter which exists in space is composed of atoms and in each atom electrons spin around a nucleus composed of protons and neutrons. Quantum Physics, which supersedes Newtonian Physics, recognises that although we see an atom as a physical structure, when Quantum Physicists wanted to find out what the atom was made out of, when they looked inside, rather than finding physical particles, they found that the atom was made out of 'vibrational' energy. This was a eureka moment when the physicists understood that matter is made out of energy, so then everything in the universe is made out of energy, and therefore it becomes important to understand that energy is very powerful in influencing what we call matter.

Now, according to Quantum Physics, matter can be influenced by the invisible energy fields and so a new kind of healing is available to us using 'energy vibration' rather than physical chemicals. And according to Bruce Lipton, PH.D, a cell biologist and an internationally recognized authority in bridging science and spirit, ***"it turns out that energy vibration as a means of communication is 100 times more efficient than trying to communicate with the body through chemistry".***(1)

We now know that all metabolic activity in the human body is controlled and regulated by what's known as the "**Quantum Energy Field**". This field is a network of electromagnetic vibrations that communicate and radiate from every cell. These electromagnetic activities register a specific frequency and each cell in our body operates at a certain frequency. Our cells network together, to keep our body in harmony.

When any kind of stressor enters the body, for example; toxins, pathogens, allergies, nutrient deficiencies, trauma, mental factors, geopathic stress, radiation or lifestyle habits, they produce erratic vibrations that impede this natural energy flow, thereby compromising to some degree the quality of one's health. If left unchecked, such stressors will over time cause a change in the body's physiology and ultimately some form of illness will develop.

Hans Selye (1907-1982), the Hungarian endocrinologist, outlined the lifecycle or flow of the disease process, where disease starts in the body as some sort of stressor. This produces an **"ALARM RESPONSE"** as the body is trying to deal with the incoming stress and this stage will provoke symptoms. If we just try to suppress the symptoms without dealing with the cause, we can interfere with healing.

As the stress continues, the body will go into an **"ADAPTATION STAGE".** In this stage symptoms will disappear as the disease progresses deeper. There is an important realisation here and it's that **"A LACK OF SYMPTONS IS NOT A SIGN OF GOOD HEALTH".** In fact you can have a serious illness and be symptom free.

When the stressor continues beyond the body's capacity to deal with it, the body enters the **"EXHAUSTION STAGE"** where the body exhausts its resources and becomes susceptible to disease and eventual death. At this stage the body is burdened with an overload of toxins and the body's organs will dysfunction and show physical damage. If the stressor continues, this last stage results in DEATH starting with cellular death → organ death → organ system death → organism death.

This disease progression can be reversed even if at the "Exhaustion Stage", once the damaging stressors are removed from the body and the natural energy flow is re-established. This is where Energy Medicine excels, by increasing the vibration or the frequency of the cells, which brings the vibrational level of the body back to its natural state of being. Energy medicine can therefore clear energetic blockages and return the body back to health by reducing the stressors that cause disease.

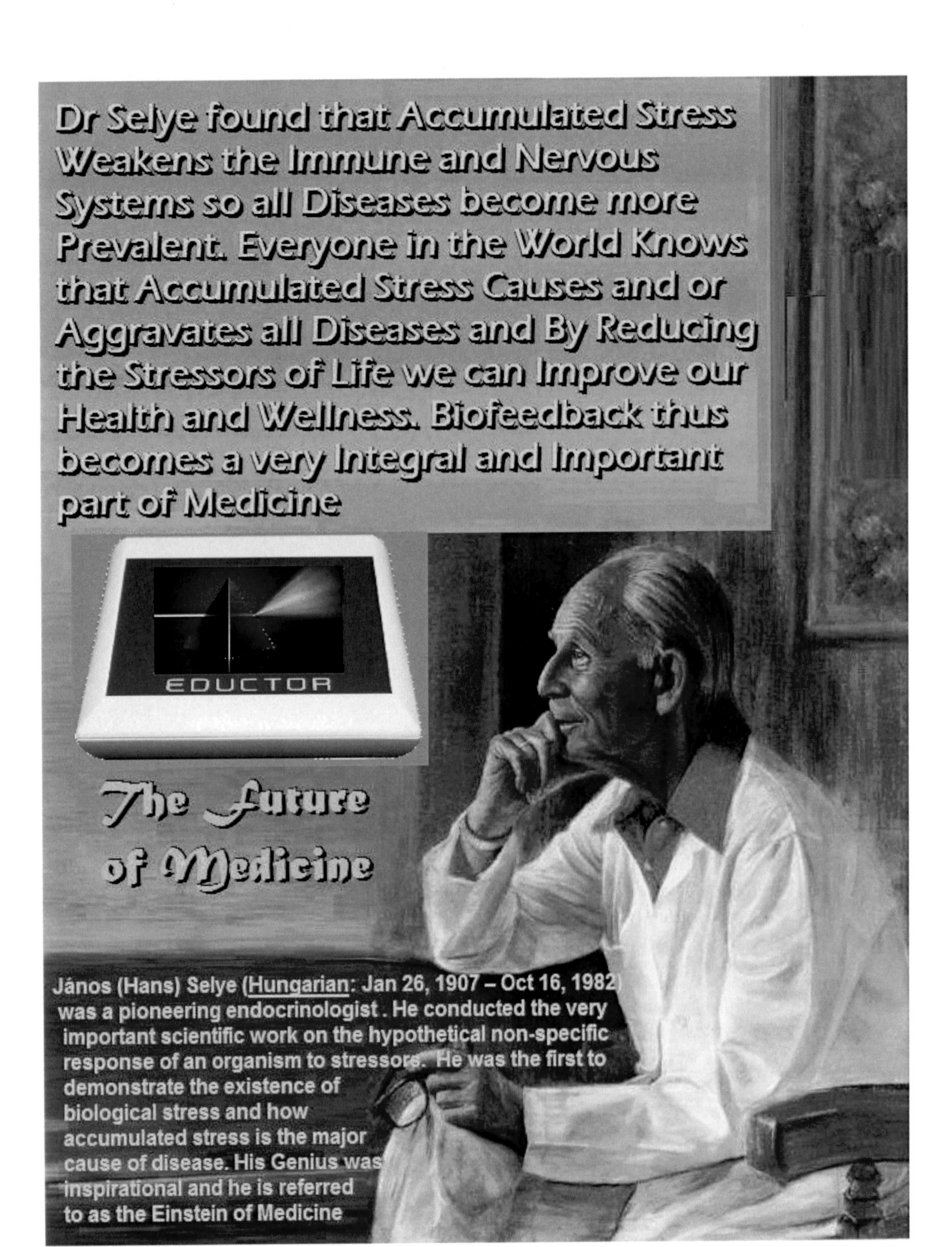
Dr Selye found that Accumulated Stress Weakens the Immune and Nervous Systems so all Diseases become more Prevalent. Everyone in the World Knows that Accumulated Stress Causes and or Aggravates all Diseases and By Reducing the Stressors of Life we can Improve our Health and Wellness. Biofeedback thus becomes a very Integral and Important part of Medicine
EDUCTOR
The Future of Medicine
János (Hans) Selye (Hungarian: Jan 26, 1907 – Oct 16, 1982) was a pioneering endocrinologist. He conducted the very important scientific work on the hypothetical non-specific response of an organism to stressors. He was the first to demonstrate the existence of biological stress and how accumulated stress is the major cause of disease. His Genius was inspirational and he is referred to as the Einstein of Medicine

THE EDUCTOR

The "EDUCTOR" is a unique biofeedback machine that can find and remove energetic stressors and blockages occurring in the body.

With this device, I am able to measure the electrical factors that cause the stress in the body and then restore these frequencies back to their correct settings. The electromagnetic waves given off by the EDUCTOR device interacts directly with the body's cells to raise their frequency, bringing them back to balance.

Stressors to the body such as viruses, bacteria, fungi, parasites, toxins, etc., all have their own specific resonant frequencies. Understanding and being able to measure all these different frequencies lets us look at a wide variety of issues affecting our health. With the Eductor we can then adjust any aberrant frequencies restoring the body to harmony and health.

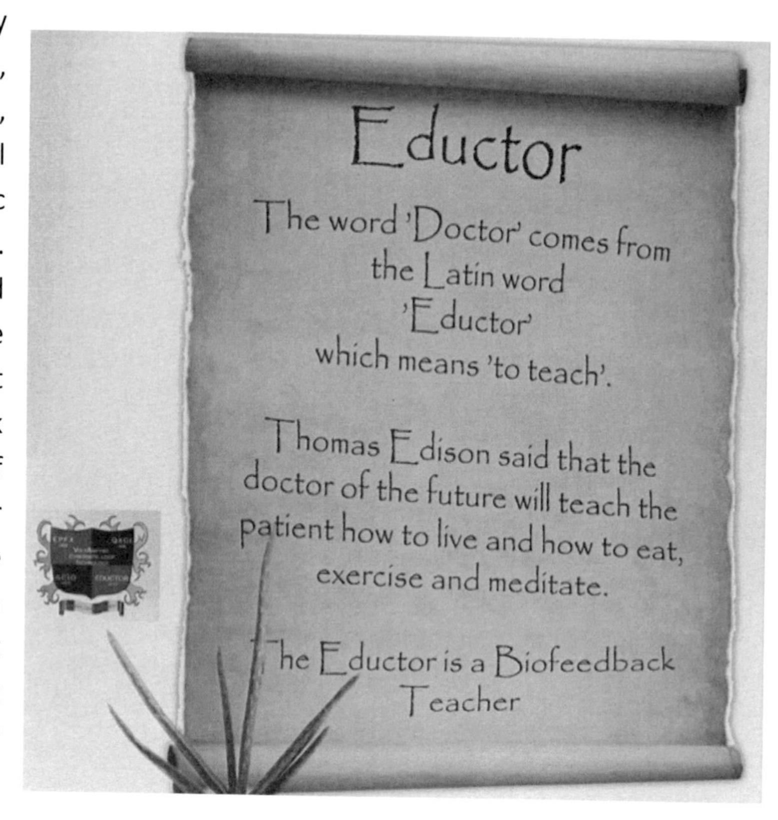

This revolutionary device is calibrated to measure over **11,000** different substance frequencies and this data offers an understanding of our body's needs, dysfunctions and weaknesses. The information obtained allows me to focus in on your energetic body, which offers a more complete view of each facet of your health. The Eductor measures multiple parameters of the human energy field including voltage, resistance, current flow, body pH, hydration and oxidation levels, along with more than 11,000 preloaded substance frequencies, and then gives effective treatment to remove any energetic imbalances and blockages within that field.

With an in-built feedback loop, the device constantly measures and mends the body's energy field through this cybernetic biofeedback loop. In other words, it sends electrical signals into the body and then measures the reactivity or response to these signals. It then sends back an alternate signal to which the body responds. In turn, your body alters its own reactivity thus creating change, for example, from imbalance to balance. The device continues to stimulate the body electric, calculate the reaction, stimulate again, re-measure, calculate, re-stimulate, and so on in a cybernetic biofeedback loop until those stressors affecting the body's energy field are nullified, thereby restoring the body to optimal health.

How is the EDUCTOR set-up?

The client is connected to the EDUCTOR by two wrist and two ankle straps as well as a head harness (see picture on next page). This provides the 2-way interface sending electromagnetic signals to the body in a safe, comfortable and non-invasive manner. The system is linked to a computer where the results can be monitored and bioenergetic therapy will be given to help restore balance.

Some of the things detected and treated by the EDUCTOR include:

- Food intolerances & Food Allergies.
- Vitamin and Mineral deficiencies
- Amino Acid and Fatty Acid deficiencies.
- Pathogens such as Viruses, Bacteria, Fungi and Parasites.
- Enzyme deficiencies
- Hormonal imbalances
- Chakra and Acupuncture Meridian blockages.

- Organ functions.
- Traumas (Physical and Mental)

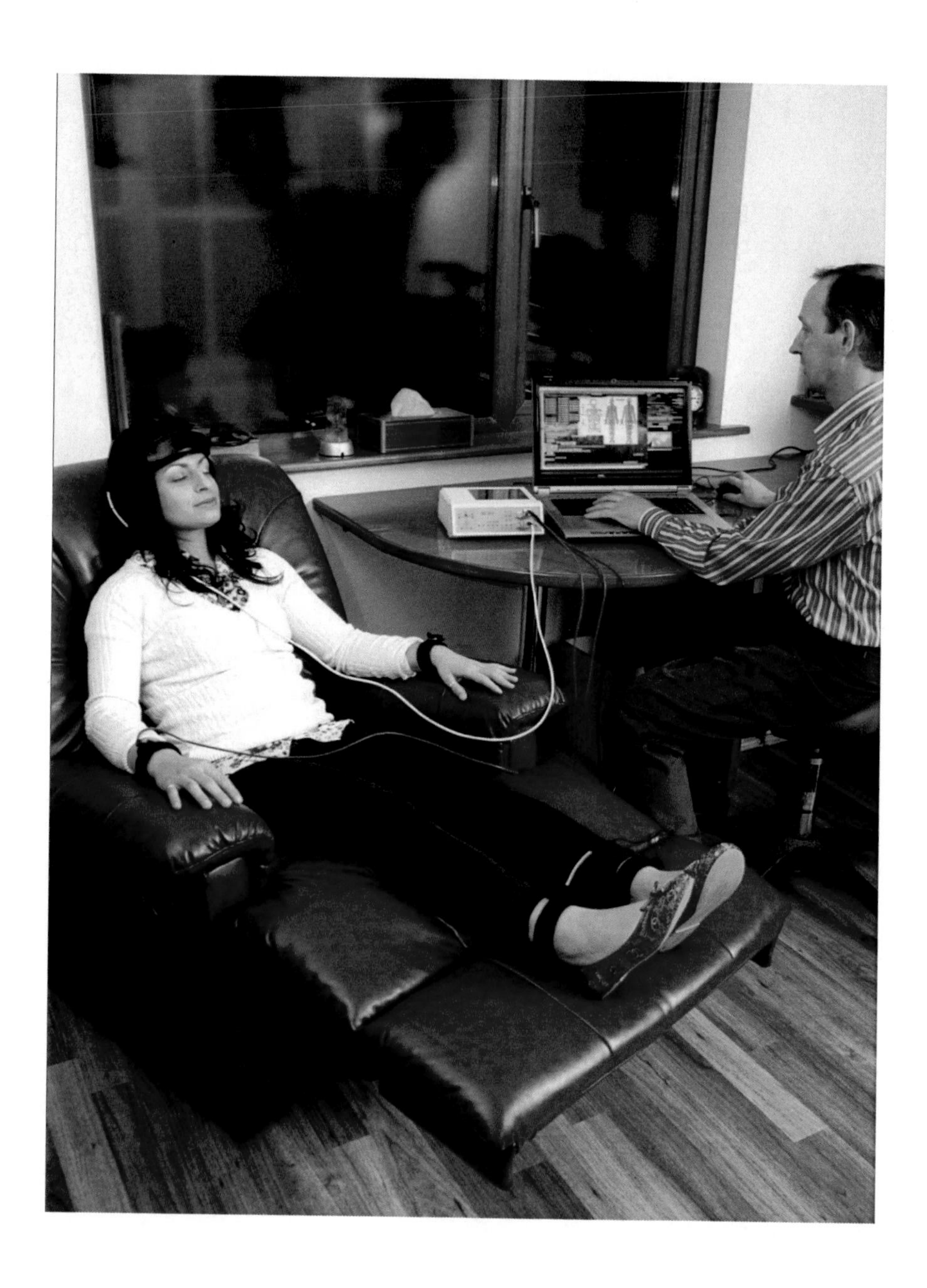

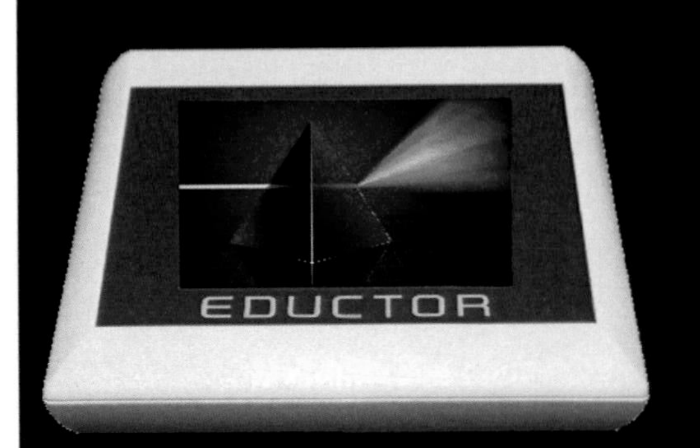

Here is a list of Conditions with Peer Reviewed Evidence the SCIO Eductor can HELP With

CONDITIONS

Research Is Proven the SCIO / Eductor can Help

- ADD/ADHD
- ADDICTION
- ANXIETY – GENERAL
- ANXIETY – PERFORMANCE
- ANXIETY – SOCIAL
- AUTISM SPECTRUM
- BRAIN INJURY / CONCUSSIONS
- CHRONIC PAIN
- DEPRESSION
- HEADACHES / MIGRAINES
- INSOMNIA
- LEARNING DIFFERENCES
- MEMORY LOSS
- OCD – OBSESSIVE COMPULSIVE DISORDER
- PANIC ATTACKS
- PTSD
- STRESS MANAGEMENT

HELP ME

Eductor Can Help

MAGNETSPACE 3D (NLS)
Health Diagnostic and Therapy System

Magnetspace 3D (NLS) is a new technology designed for both investigation and treatment of the human body. It is the latest and most precise **Non Linear Diagnostic System (NLS)** that can accurately test the condition of all the body systems and organs right down to the cellular level. Not only can you see 3D images of the results projected onto a screen, the system can also identify the origins of any disease process, whether it was due to viruses, microbes, fungi, parasites, allergies or other factors. In addition, this remarkable system also has an inbuilt "**Repair Treatment**" function that sends out harmonizing frequencies to aid in the repair of damaged tissues and organs.

Principles of Operation of Non Linear (NLS) Diagnostic Systems Technology

NLS devices are based on the study of ***magnetic 'torsion fields'*** created within biological bodies. These pioneering devices were first researched and developed in Russia in the early 1990's by researchers from the Institute of Practical Psychophysics. The basic idea behind the development of this

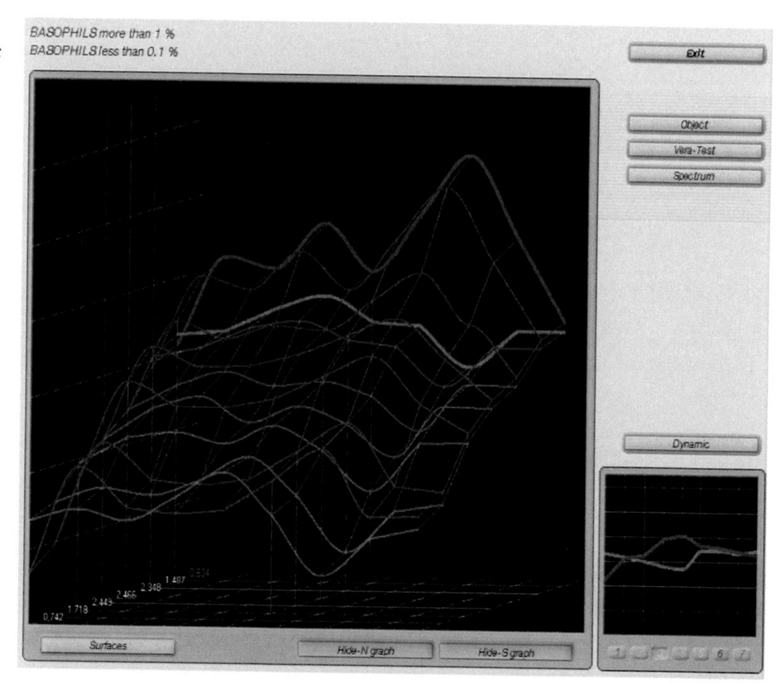

equipment was the hypothesis that the human body's energy field has an electromagnetic (torsion field) informational framework, capable of responding to external frequency emissions. Based on this understanding, the researchers from the Institute of Practical Psychophysics created the first NLS research equipment allowing them to monitor the physical condition of the body through changes in the wave characteristics of the body's cells, tissues and organs.

The NLS device evaluates an organ's condition based on the resonant amplification of the investigated organ's wave emission. It does this with the aid of special trigger sensors connected to a resonance chamber that can amplify and read these frequency parameters.

NLS Analysis System

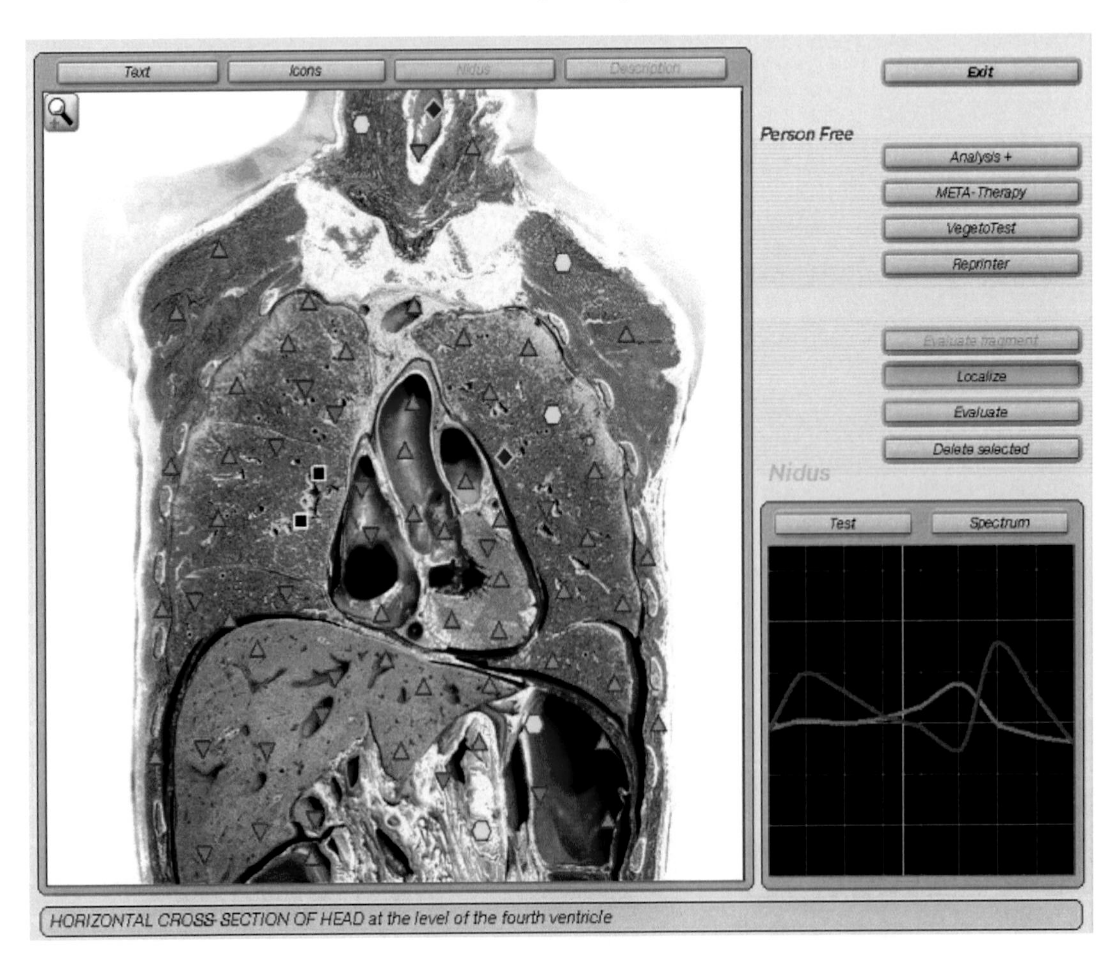

Each organ and each cell have their own unique frequency oscillations, which are stored in the computer memory of the NLS device. Also stored in the computer memory are the frequency oscillations of all known diseases or pathological processes, as they too, have their unique wave characteristics.

During a test, the NLS device measures all the frequency characteristics of the body's cells, tissues and organs, and compares them by magnitude of spectral similarity with the computer's reference processes (i.e. - against healthy and pathologically changed tissues, including infectious agents) to reveal the closest pathological process or a tendency to its development.

The main advantages of NLS diagnostics lies in the principle of the method been very sensitive to the dynamics of pathological changes and thus can detect a tendency to an illness or disease at an early stage when they are not yet apparent at tissue level.

Magnetspace 3D (NLS) – How it works

The Magnetspace 3D (NLS) is based on the spectral analysis of the magnetic torsion fields created by the body's tissues and organs. These electromagnetic vibrations, which contain all the information about the state of the body's health is delivered to the brain in frequency format. The Magnetspace 3D device uses a resonance chamber to amplify these frequency vibrations that are picked up by means of special trigger sensors, which are shaped as headphones and placed over the ears.

The special software incorporated into this system is able to obtain the incoming data, decode it and display the results on a computer screen in the form of three dimensional (3D) models of the body's tissues and organs.

Varying degrees of tissue and organ dysfunction or damage are highlighted according to their actual condition. All tissues and organs that have been identified as problematic can then be examined in greater detail to reveal the foci of contamination at the required perspective. For instance, the Magnetspace 3D can perform a series of vertical and horizontal slices through any tissue or organ, increasing the magnification right down to the cellular level, to obtain a clearer and more detailed picture of the organ in question. With this feature, it can determine how much the body is burdened by various toxins, whether it's from viral, bacterial, fungal, parasitic or other factors.

The Magnetspace 3D device also has the capacity to generate a series of electromagnetic harmonizing fields that can correct any aberrant frequency oscillations of stressed or diseased tissue, bringing the biochemical activity of these tissues to a level that corresponds to normal tissue function. In other words it can correct defects and pathologies in organs and body cells.

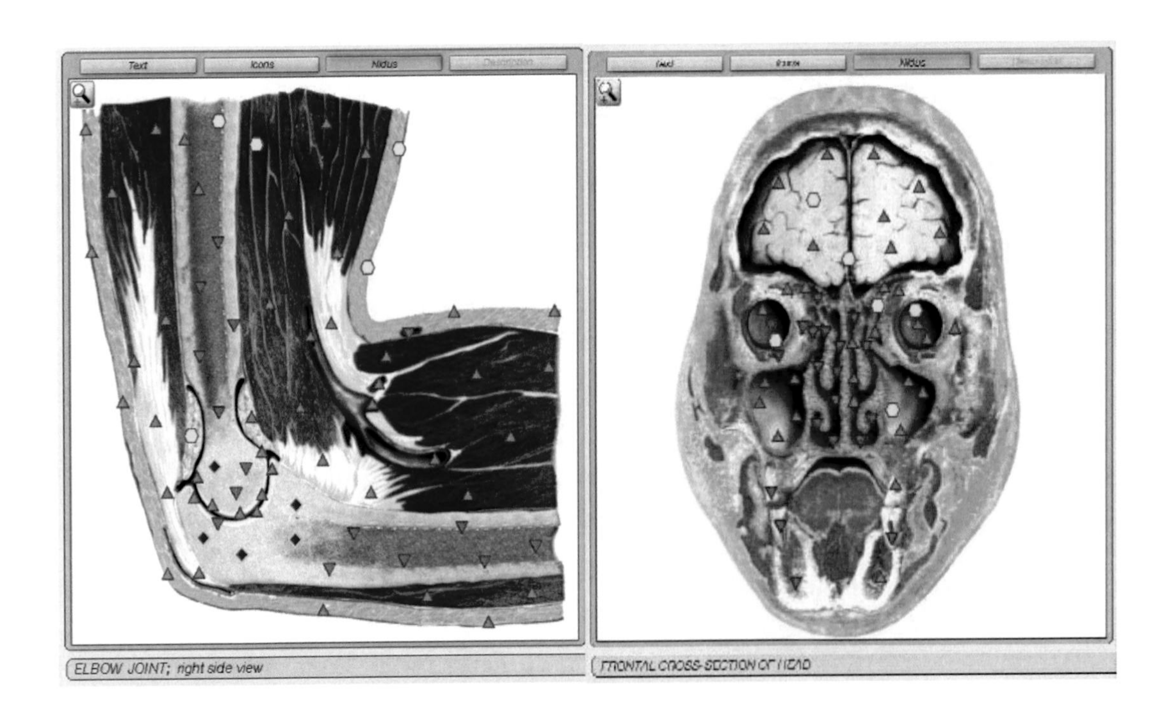

Advantages of Magnetspace 3D (NLS)

- Finds the hidden causes behind the symptoms
- Makes disorders qualitatively and quantitatively visible
- A comparative analysis between before and after therapy is shown
- Ideal as a prevention therapy as it recognises the disorder in its early form
- Accurately tests for pollutants and other burdens
- Finds allergies and food intolerances and treats them with bio-resonance
- Calculates in advance the efficiency of a remedy
- Sends out harmonizing frequencies with the inbuilt META Therapy function

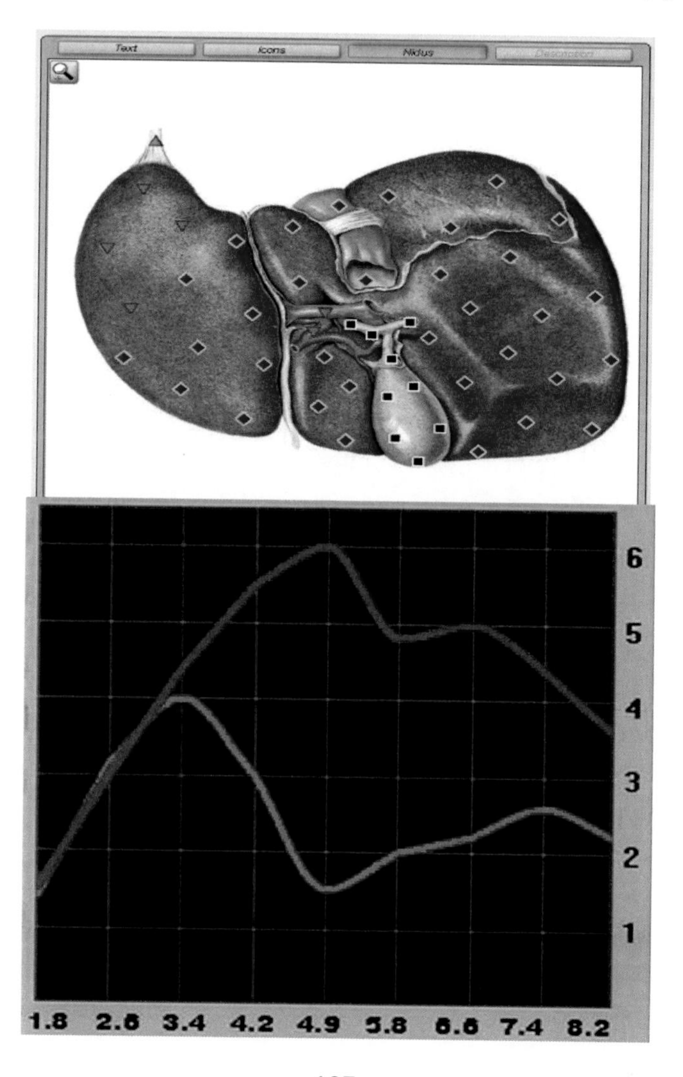

Chapter 12

LAST WORD

"If you don't take care of your body, where will you live" – Author Unknown

One of the themes running through this book has been the simple truth: that the generation of disease is primarily due to our **"inverted way of eating and living"** instead of being the result of our genetics or outside uncontrollable events of nature.

It never ceases to amaze me that some people can live their entire lives in denial about their health. A prime characteristic of human nature is to assume that bad things only happen to other people. And so with this cavalier attitude many of us smoke cigarettes, gorge ourselves on too much junk food, drink alcohol excessively, and rarely exercise, thinking these things will not harm us. Then when we do inevitably get sick, our first thought is to run to our doctor to fix us. And the doctor goes: Okay, here's a pill for your blood pressure, and here's a pill for your cholesterol, and here's a pill for your back pain, and I'll see you in a month and we'll see if you're maintaining your disease. And that's what doctors do! – they maintain a person's illness. They are not making them better - And that's not okay! They are supposed to return people to a state of optimal health, or as close as possible to; that is their job. The word Doctor means "to teach". Why aren't they teaching their patients how to turn their health around?

When the doctor treats a sick person they invariably give a medicine that attempts to overpower the symptoms that accompany disease. So if you've been diagnosed with arthritis, you are given anti-inflammatory and pain-relieving medicines; heartburn or indigestion is relived with antacids; infections are treated with antibiotics; high temperatures with antipyretics and headaches are relieved with painkillers. This reductionist approach to disease leads to a dead end in treatment because these medicines are not curative. Have you ever heard of anyone being cured of their high blood pressure, their diabetes or their arthritis with allopathic medicine? No! That's because drugs can only offer management of the symptoms of disease through suppressive means.

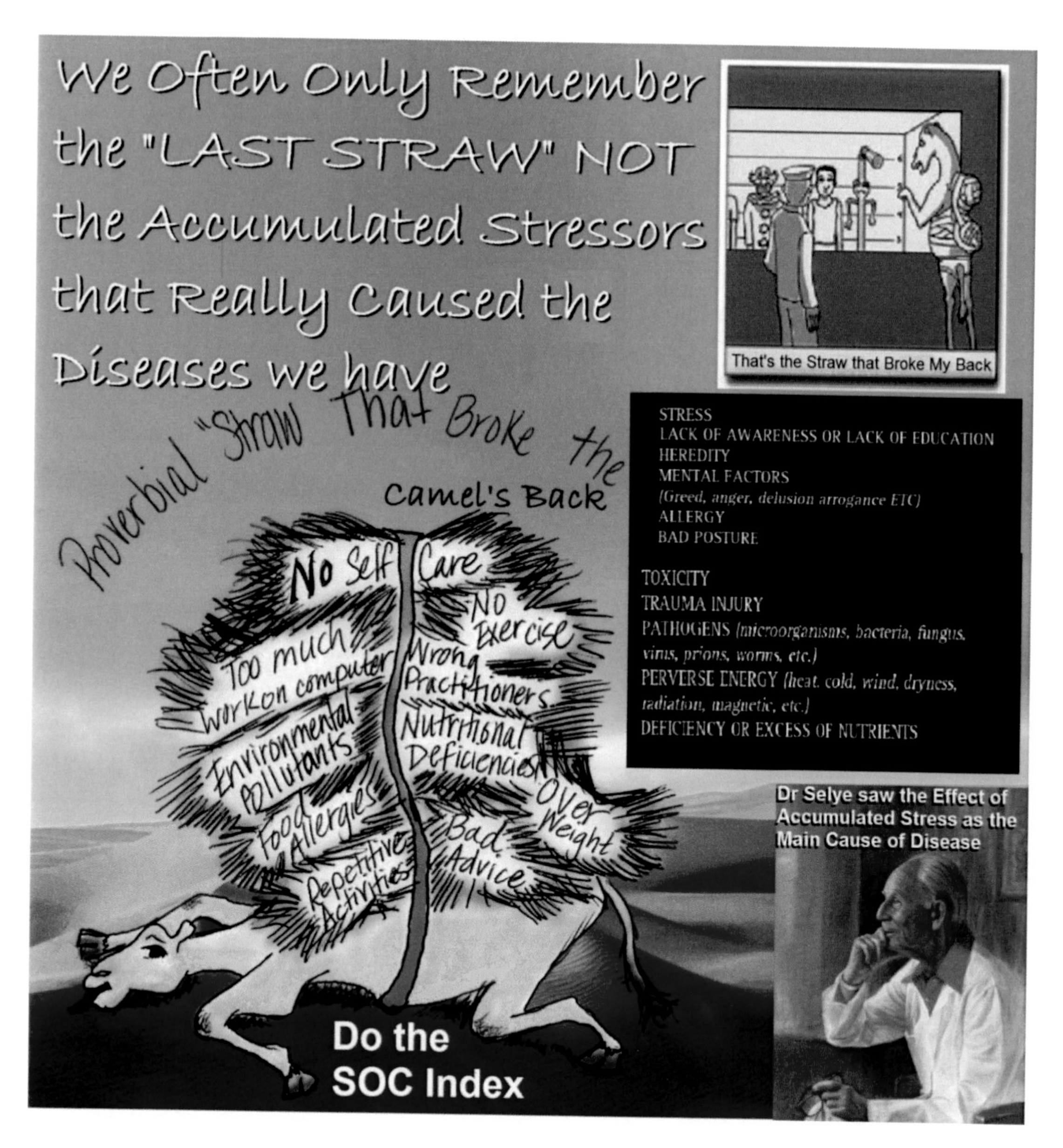

Most drugs merely work to minimize the symptoms but don't address the fundamental causes of disease. The effect is to create a plethora of side-effects and complications, which results in yet more need of medical intervention.

Even though most doctors recognize the need to deal with the underlying causes of illness, their capacity to do so is limited by their lack of understanding of the fundamental causes of disease. However, on the other hand, if one were to apply the principles of naturopathic medicine, their disease process can then be easily reversed when they stop eating foods that hurt their bodies and put into practice the fundamental elements of life and health in necessary measure. These fundamental elements are: proper diet, pure water, fresh air and sunlight, adequate sleep and exercise, positive mental outlook and emotional harmony.

The simple but surprising truth of the matter is that the elimination of most diseases is easy. It is a "natural" law that how well we live, how much health and vitality we have, and how well we will feel in the future depends totally on us. It all boils down to one thing: **"our choices!"** Our present and future health depends on the choices we now make. Our choices so far, have led to our self-induced pain and disease states. That needn't be the case any longer. New health-promoting choices can create a new you. Change your choices and you will change your health and your life for the better forever.

Our understanding of health and disease has been framed by 100 years of biomedical hegemony. Allopathic medicine has formulated the biomedical model of disease and so, has been able to shape society's beliefs about ill health and how it should be managed.

We are led to believe that sickness and chronic disease are inevitable, that we were most likely cursed at birth by some mysterious "bad" gene, or that disease is simply a function of aging. We mistakenly believe that the older we get, the more our bodies must deteriorate.

The medical profession tries to scare people into thinking that they can't really do anything to control their own disease once it takes hold. The general public have been conditioned to believe that the reason they are sick is mostly because of "bad" genes: that chronic diseases such as arthritis, Alzheimer's, auto-immune conditions, depression, diabetes, heart disease, hypothyroidism, multiple sclerosis, osteoporosis, Parkinson's, etc., etc., are mostly the result of poor genetics.

There are a few diseases that are in fact genetic in nature. They are all congenital, which means that they happen to the developing foetus while in the mother's womb. Down's syndrome, Cystic fibrosis and Cleft lip/palate are three common genetic diseases. What's not generally known is that the genes that code for these diseases gets **'turned on'** in the absence of a particular nutrient in the pregnant mother. For instance: the gene that expresses Down's syndrome becomes active if the mother is deficient in zinc; Cystic fibrosis is caused by a deficiency in selenium and Cleft lip/palate is caused by not enough vitamin B12 in the mother during pregnancy.(57)

Their biomedical model approach tends to equate illness and disease as the result of a biological process in which something malfunctions in the body and therefore they must intervene to fix the malfunction with drugs or surgery.

Such an approach to disease can be regarded as ***reactive*** rather than ***proactive*** in nature. Allopathic medicine is primarily focused upon the treatment of disease and hence upon alleviating the symptoms of illness and not upon the maintenance of health or upon stimulating the body's own innate healing processes.

Certainly there have been triumphs in surgery and in the immediate treatment of acute infectious illnesses, but the same cannot be said for chronic and degenerative diseases. The reason why allopathic medicine has had very limited or no success in treating chronic disease is because of its very narrow approach to health care. Its eternal search for "magic bullets" to eliminate disease ignores the many ways we create disease in the first place; ways I have outlined in great detail throughout this book. That's why to date; modern medicine has not discovered "cures" for the many diseases of affluence. Their prescribed medicines never treat the underlying causes of illness, drug treatments simply cover up the symptoms of disease only.....

Optimal health and illness can be illustrated as being at the opposite ends of a *wellness continuum*. There are many segments between these two extremes and illness does not come on suddenly without several steps being crossed first. This is especially the case with all chronic degenerative conditions.

You don't for instance; wake up one morning suffering from arthritic pain. The arthritic pain came on slowly over time as your body progressively succumbs to the effects of its toxic state. Then when the pain becomes unbearable you resort to taking painkillers, however the cause of the pain is left unchanged. Pain relief can be fast while on painkillers but the pain will keep returning until something more is done about the issue.

Getting your body back to a state of optimal health, especially if you are starting from the other end of the wellness continuum takes time because a process of healing is involved. To help this process there are a number of very simple, clear and inexpensive steps you can take to improve your health. If you have any health challenges or if you simply want to maintain the best of health, my experience of treating thousands of people over the last fifteen years has shown that the most important things you can do are:

- Eat organic and whole natural foods
- Keep your body adequately hydrated with clean water
- Cut out sugar by eliminating from your diet all foods that contain added sugar.
- Eat the right fats (i.e. cold water fish, fish oils, olive oil, coconut oil, butter)
- Avoid toxic environments and reduce toxins in the diet by eating organic.
- Avoid nutrient robbers such as all junk foods.
- Stop smoking and reduce alcohol intake to safe levels.
- Take nutritional supplements to fill the nutrient void in your diet.
- Take herbal medicines appropriate to your condition.
- Get regular sunlight exposure.

- Exercise regularly.
- Take time for some recreational activity and also get plenty of sleep.
- And finally, be aware of mental and emotional factors that influence your habits and your health.

No matter where you are on the continuum of health to illness, you can always reverse it one step at a time. Even if you are on death's door and taking a dozen or more medications, you can still find a new level of health by turning to good nutrition, along with all the things I just suggested. **You too,** can turn your life around; people do it all the time.

It is a sure process. You take it one step at a time with your choices. You make a new choice each day that you get up. You say today I am no longer going to drink soft drinks, or today I am no longer going to allow sugar and artificial sweeteners in my diet, or I am going to give up eating nutrient-deficient white bread along with biscuits and cakes because I know how terrible those foods are for my health. You could say anything along those lines.

You could say, today I am going to start drinking and eating superfoods for breakfast every day, or today I am going to start doing the nutritional supplementation programme that I know is good for me. Today I am going to make a change for the better, and when you do that one step at a time, you take control of your health journey from that point forward. It all comes down to you and the choices you make.

Here is an optimistic and totally realistic idea to carry with you *"most health problems are reversible!"* You need only, to start making the right choices.

Live long in Health

John Byrne

THE HISTORY OF MEDICINE

2000 B.C. - HERE, EAT THIS ROOT.

DRINK THIS JUICE

1000 A.D. - THAT ROOT IS HEATHEN.

HERE, SAY THIS PRAYER.

1850 A.D. - THAT PRAYER IS SUPERSTITION.

HERE, DRINK THIS POTION.

1940 A.D. - THAT POTION IS SNAKE OIL.

HERE, SWALLOW THIS PILL.

1985. A.D. - THAT PILL IS INEFFECTIVE.

HERE, TAKE THIS *SYNTHETIC DRUG*

2011 A.D. - THAT *SYNTHETIC DRUG DON'T WORK*

HERE, EAT THIS ROOT.

DON'T EAT SYNTHETICS, DRINK THIS JUICE

SAY THIS PRAYER.

APPENDIX 1

GUIDELINES FOR HEALTHY EATING

ON RISING: (i.e. Before Breakfast)

Immediately upon waking each day, choice of:

- Squeeze about ½ to 1 full lemon (depending on the size of the lemon) into a full glass of lukewarm water
- One tablespoon of apple cider vinegar in full glass of warm water
- Small glass of freshly squeezed grapefruit juice.

- Any of the above substances neutralises body acidity, aids in the elimination of toxins, improves your digestion, stimulates your metabolism and boosts your energy for the day.

BREAKFAST

Choose only one of the following breakfast suggestions each day. For variety and food rotation (i.e. try to avoid eating the same foods every day), choose a different breakfast choice each day.

- Scrambled egg with tomato, sautéed onions and mushrooms.
- A poached or soft boiled egg with wholemeal toast or buckwheat/rye bread.
- Pinhead oatmeal porridge with raisins and Chia Bia seeds. Serve with choice of rice milk, soya milk, coconut milk, sesame milk or almond milk.
- Choice of "organic" Weetabix, cornflakes, or rice bubbles (all low in sugar) mixed with organic goat's milk or one of the above milks.
- Millet or Buckwheat porridge with raisins and almonds.
- Rice cakes with almond, cashew or hazelnut butter.

- Fresh seasonal fruit (eat melons alone)
- Non-sweetened muesli, preferably home-made (health food stores have a good selection).
- Organic yoghurt.
- Smoothies made with coconut milk, can add organic yoghurt, fruit, nuts, lecithin, flaxseeds or chia bia seeds.
- Organic baked beans on wholemeal toast (use a variety of grains i.e.: wheat, rye, corn, buckwheat, spelt).

LUNCH/DINNER

Ideally, this should be the main meal of the day when animal or vegetarian protein is consumed. Having your protein at lunchtime gives your body plenty of time to properly digest it before going to bed. A heavy protein meal in the evening is not good for sleep or your digestive system.

- Fish, i.e. salmon, mackerel, herring, tuna, sardines, trout, (all high in Omega 3 fatty acids) with salad or vegetables. N.B. Try to eat these fish two or three times per week.
- Roast beef, or lean beef fillet or lamb cutlet, T-bone steak with potato and vegetables (limit to once per week).
- A hearty soup, like lentil or bean, with whole grain bread and a salad.
- Slices of either chicken or turkey breast, or tuna or egg or sardines with salad.
- Caesar salad with a little cottage cheese.
- Pasta dishes, e.g. Penne, Carbonara, Ravioli, Fettuccine, (can be made with chicken, seafood or vegetables).
- Bean and vegetable casserole with colcannon (mashed potatoes, cabbage, onion, milk and butter).
- Stir fry veggies and Tofu or Tempeh or chicken or fish with garlic, spices and brown rice. (Tofu can be marinated in Shoyu or Tamari sauce with added garlic and spices for added flavour).
- Tuna, chicken, turkey or egg salad sandwich (brown bread only) with soup.

- Rice or spelt bread and baked beans with salad.
- Broccoli, Goats cheese, eggplant, potato and chickpea salad.
- Vegetable omelette with choice of bread.

EVENING MEAL (SUPPER)

Refrain from eating a large meal at the end of the day. Ideally your evening meal should be light and easy to digest and consist mostly of carbohydrates. (Eating carbohydrates in the evening promotes better sleep. You will also sleep more soundly if you avoid stimulating drinks such as tea and coffee).

- Stuffed baked potato (with vegetables only; no protein with evening meal i.e. no cheese, eggs or meats).
- Vegetable based soup with wholegrain bread.
- Corn on the cob with vegetables or garden salad.
- Mushroom and spinach risotto (1tbsp olive oil, 25 g butter, 1 chopped onion, 140g of sliced chestnut mushrooms, garlic clove, 140g arboria rice, 100g spinach, 4 chopped sundried tomatoes, some chopped parsley, 500ml vegetable stock, 150ml dry white wine) served with green salad.
- Banana bread sandwich with chamomile tea.
- Vegetable pie or pasta salad.
- Steamed or sautéed vegetable with brown rice or millet.
- Tomato, corn and avocado salad mixed with chopped scallions and a salad dressing made from lime or lemon juice, safflower or flaxseed oil and seasoned with sea salt and ground pepper.
- Hummus and roasted veggie tortilla wrap (handful of your favourite vegetable, e.g. spinach, tomatoes, zucchini), roast veggies for 30 minutes at 200^{0}C with the olive oil, crushed garlic, salt and pepper. Spread the hummus over the soft tortilla shell, add the roasted veggies roll it up and bake for 10 minutes.
- Vegetarian filled red peppers (2 red pepper halves filled with arboria rice, courgettes, mushrooms, onions in tomato sauce sprinkled with grated cheese).

- Grilled asparagus and red onions with salad dressing served with potatoes.

SNACKS

If you tend to get hungry before or between meals you can have one of the following snacks:

- Nuts and seeds (small handful) or dried fruit.
- Wholemeal fruit muffins.
- Wholegrain or rice crackers with nut butter (almond, cashew, hazelnut, etc.).
- Carrot and celery sticks with hummus or guacamole dip.
- Rice cakes with avocado, tomato and sea salt.
- Rice or coconut smoothies with fresh fruit.
- Unsweetened organic yoghurt or soya yoghurt.
- Tahini and honey (mixed) on rice cakes.

OTHER SUGGESTIONS TO CONSIDER

- Eat at the right time. Eat breakfast within one to two hours of rising, lunch/dinner approximately four to five hours later, and super within six hours of lunch. Eating properly increased your metabolism, which burns more calories.
- Drink plenty of filtered water throughout the day, not too much with meals though.
- Rotate foods, i.e. try to avoid eating the same foods every day, use as much variety as possible.
- Wherever possible, use organically grown fruit, vegetables and meats.
- Buy whole, fresh foods only, instead of canned, packaged and processed food.
- Use only organic olive and coconut oils in cooking (safe at high temperature).
- Minimise your intake of tea and coffee and replace with herbal teas, .ie. fennel, peppermint, green tea, chamomile, etc.

APPENDIX 2

ANIT-INFLAMMATORY NUTRITIONAL PROGRAMME

Levels of inflammation can be reduced in the body by incorporating certain dietary guidelines. Foods that are high in saturated and hydrogenated fats, sugars, refined carbohydrates, yeast, caffeine, alcohol, artificial colours, flavours and preservatives, need to be avoided as they promote inflammation in the body. Approximately 75% to 80% of your dietary intake should consist of the following anti-inflammatory foods:

- **Vegetables:** unlimited amounts of preferably organic vegetables should be eaten daily. It is best to limit the nightshade vegetables (i.e. potatoes, chillies, tomatoes, eggplant and peppers) which have a chemical alkaloid called solanine that may trigger inflammation in some individuals.
- **Fruit**: All fruit (watch out for oranges as they can aggravate arthritic conditions).
- **Salads:** Unlimited amounts of green leafy salads, fresh sprouts and grated raw vegetables should be eaten daily.
- **Grains:** Rice, buckwheat, oats, rye, millet, corn and quinoa can be used freely (soak the grains overnight and cook with a pinch of sea salt to aid digestion. Reduce or avoid wheat and all wheat products as they are promoters of inflammation.
- **Fish:** Salmon, mackerel, herring, tuna, trout, sardines and anchovies are cold water fish that contain omega-3 oils with anti-inflammatory components. Eat a selection of these fish at least 3 times per week.
- **Beans:** Chickpeas, kidney, butter, cannellini, haricot, pinto, mung, broad, aduki, black-eyed beans, lentils and peas. A small piece of kombu sea weed can be added while soaking overnight to assist digestion and reduce gas

production.

- **Nuts & Seeds:** A small handful daily from the following: walnuts, almonds, brazil nuts, cashews, hazelnuts, flaxseed, sunflower seeds, pumpkin seeds, chia bia seeds and sesame seeds.
- **Oils:** olive and coconut oil in salads and for cooking. Sesame, flax and cod liver oil (not for cooking).
- **Beverages:** Pure water, spring or filtered is best. Herbal teas. Healthful green drinks can be made from powdered forms of wheatgrass, spirulina, barley grass and chlorella.
- **Spices:** The best anti-inflammatory spices are turmeric, ginger, garlic thyme, rosemary, bay leaves, oregano, and black pepper.

FOODS TO REDUCE OR AVOID

You should limit your consumption of the following pro-inflammatory foods to no more than 20% to 25% of your dietary intake.

- **Meats:** Red meat, lamb, pork, ham, bacon, organ meats, sausages and processed luncheon meats. Replace with oily fish, organic chicken and vegetarian protein (i.e. beans, legumes, tofu, tempeh).
- **Dairy:** Cow's milk, hard cheeses, cream, sour cream, ice-cream, sweetened yoghurts and artificial butters. (Try rice milk, sesame seed milk, almond or oat milk to replace. Soft cheeses like cottage or ricotta are better alternatives. Organic yoghurts and goat's yoghurt are preferable).
- **Fats:** Animal fats, lard, shortening, fried foods, junk foods, fast-food, takeaways, vegetable oils such as corn, soya, canola, safflower and peanut oils; margarine and most commercial artificial butters as well as most commercial salad dressings. All these products contain inflammatory promoters.
- **Shellfish:** Prawns, crabs and lobster (are pro-inflammatory). Keep with the cold water oily fish including scallops as the better alternatives.
- **Sugar:** White, brown, honey, jams, cakes, biscuits, pastries, chocolate,

sweets, canned fruits, desserts, ice-cream and commercial breakfast cereals are all full of sugar. Use organic molasses to substitute.

- **Yeast:** Avoid yeast breads and yeast extracts such as Bovril, Marmite and Vegemite. The better brands to eat are rice, buckwheat, rye and corn breads.
- **Artificial Food Additives:** Aspartame; monosodium glutamate (MSG) along with a myriad of preservatives, flavourings, colourings, etc., that are found in processed and packaged foods. If you order Chinese food make sure you've the option to ask for no MSG.
- **Drinks:** Drink mostly filtered water, herbal teas and healthful green drinks, not soft drinks, fruit juices, alcohol or caffeinated beverages.

APPENDIX 3

ANIT-CANDIDA DIETARY PROGRAMME

This diet is based on the principle that fermented foods and sugary foods encourage Candida to grow. You will need to stop feeding the candida with these foods for a period of three months whilst making sure that the friendly bacteria in the gut gets nurtured and well fed in order to bring the candida back under control.

FOODS TO AVOID FOR A 3 MONTH PERIOD:

Foods containing sugar and refined carbohydrates. This includes:

- White and brown sugar
- Honey, glucose, syrups, liquors, molasses
- All confectionary products including cakes, biscuits, croissants and pastries.
- All soft drinks and fruit juices.
- Chocolate and other sweets.
- White flour products, white rice.
- Hidden sugars in processed foods.
- All fresh or dried fruit including jams for the first month. During the second and third month, you are allowed small amounts of pawpaw, pineapple, kiwifruit, mango, bananas, honeydew melon, grapefruit, apples, pears.

YEAST CONTAINING (FERMENTED) FOODS AND MOULD-CONTAMINATED FOODS INCLUDING:

- Commercial brands, rolls, pizzas, muffins, biscuits and cakes.
- Dairy products, i.e. cow's milk, cheese, yoghurt, cream, buttermilk, ice-cream.
- Yeast extract, (Bovril, Vegemite, Marmite, etc.).
- All alcoholic drinks – (beer, wine, cider, spirits, etc.).

- Fermented foods such as tofu, tempeh, quorn and miso.
- All types of mushrooms.
- All vinegars, commercial sauces, mayonnaise, soy sauce, mustard, salad dressings.
- Processed meats such as sausage, salami, ham, pepperoni.
- Peanuts, pistachios or old nuts and seeds.
- Black tea and coffee
- Vitamin B-Complex and any health products containing brewer's yeast.

FOODS THAT YOU CAN EAT INCLUDE THE FOLLOWING:

- All vegetables, steamed, cooked or stir-fried; avoid eating them raw.
- Meats including lean meat, chicken, turkey, lamb and fresh fish (organic if possible).
- Eggs and goat's milk, goat's cheese and yoghurt, butter, coconut milk, rice cakes.
- Buckwheat bread, rice and corn breads, corn tortillas, soda bread (check for buttermilk).
- Cereals: rice flakes, corn puffs, millet flakes, buckwheat flakes.
- Pastas: rice, corn, buckwheat.
- Legumes: beans, peas, lentils, chickpeas.
- Grains: Quinoa, buckwheat, millet and brown rice.
- Fresh nuts and seeds (except peanuts and pistachios).
- Oils: Olive, coconut, flaxseed, sesame, avocado (store opened bottles in fridge).
- Herbal teas especially Pau D'arco and Fennel; filtered water with a squeeze of lemon juice; diluted vegetable juices.
- Spreads: avocado, guacamole, hummus, tahini.

ANTI-CANDIDA DIET SUGGESTIONS

Breakfast

- Rice flakes, sugar free corn flakes, or millet flake cereal with coconut milk or goat's milk.
- Boiled egg or poached or scrambled egg on buckwheat or corn bread.
- Tahini on rice cakes sprinkled with sunflower seed.

Morning & Evening Snack

- Hazelnut, almond or other nut butter (not peanut or pistachio) on rice bread.
- ½ cup of fresh nuts and seeds.
- Guacamole (avocado dip) with tortilla chips or spread over rice bread.
- Sardine pate (canned sardines, garlic clove, knob of butter, chopped parsley & juice of lemon blended) served on rice crackers.
- Tahini or hummus on rice toast sprinkled with seeds.
- Hummus dip with carrot and celery sticks
- Herbal tea with rice cakes

Lunch

- Grilled chicken (marinated overnight in olive oil, lemon juice, chopped onion, crushed garlic clove, paprika and black pepper), served with salad and rice.
- Tuna fish cakes (made with mashed potatoes, chopped parsley and black pepper) served with salad.
- Stir fry of onions, garlic and vegetables with buckwheat pasta.
- Salad sandwich with home-made hummus (chickpeas, lemon juice, garlic and tahini).
- Salmon and lentil salad.
- Roasted corn and bean salad (lima beans, kidney beans, onions, garlic,

coriander, sea salt, pepper, olive oil).

- Salad with chicken breast and rice.
- Stir-fry vegetables with lean beef mince and rice noodles.

Dinner

- Brown rice and split pea vegetable soup.
- Avocado and cucumber soup.
- Veggies and goat's cheese.
- Baked chicken and vegetables
- Asparagus and anchovies with buckwheat noodles.
- Mince patties on rice bread with salad.
- Veggie-burger (mash vegetables and combine with cooked rice and an egg to form patties) with salad on corn or rice bread.
- Fillet of fresh fish with salad (linseed oil and lemon juice dressing) on vegetables.
- Poached mackerel fillet in coconut cream. Serve on a bed of rice with salad.
- Grilled lime chicken breast with salad (juice of 2 limes, 3 garlic cloves, 2 chillies, 1 tbsp. olive oil, salt & pepper).

APPENDIX 4

LOW REACTIVE ELIMINATION DIET

The purpose of this diet is to remove the most common food allergens and chemical sensitivities for a period of three weeks followed by a challenge phase to identify any food allergies and chemical sensitivities.

This diet is designed to eliminate:

- Dairy products (milk, cheese, cream, yoghurt, ice-cream, kefir).
- Gluten containing foods (wheat, rye, oats, barley) and any foods containing them, e.g. couscous, tabbouleh, beer, ketchup.
- Nightshade vegetables (potato, tomato, artichoke, peppers, egg plant).
- Yeast and mould containing foods.
- Eggs and foods containing egg.
- Soya products including tofu, tempeh, miso, soya sauce, soya milk, tamari.
- Chocolate, sugar, caffeine.
- All alcohol.
- Shell fish.
- High salicylate foods (apricots, cherries, raspberries, strawberries, plums, dates, all dried fruits, orange, pineapple, blueberries, cranberry (See page 36).
- Preservatives (nitrates, metabisulphite).
- Flavour enhancers such as MSG, aspartame.
- High amine foods containing histamines, tyranine, or serotonin (See page 36).

FOODS YOU CAN EAT ON THE LOW REACTIVE ELIMINATION DIET:

- Chicken, turkey, lamb, beef, veal, fish, scallops.
- Grains: rice, millet, quinoa.

- Vegetables: sweet potatoes, carrots, pumpkin cabbage, spinach, cauliflower, brussel sprouts, leek, zucchini, beetroot, bean shoots, spring onion, lettuce, cucumber, garlic.
- Fruits: pears, bananas, apples, mango, avocado, pawpaw, rock melon.
- Legumes & Nuts: lentils, chickpeas, cashews, green beans, peas, mung beans.
- Cooking condiments including butter, salt, olive oil, coconut oil, pepper, and fresh culinary herbs.
- Drinks: purified water, rice milk, coconut milk, natural lemonade, tea and coffee if you can't live without.

LOW REACTIVE ELIMINATION DIET MENU PLAN

The following is an example of a low reactive elimination diet. Simply eat these foods on the suggested days for a period of three weeks, (slight modifications can be made so long as none of the forbidden foods are consumed).

As your body clears during this elimination phase, you could experience a temporary worsening of symptoms. These may include headaches, brain fog, skin rash, bloating, flatulence, fatigue or constipation. Such symptoms are a common part of the clearing process and should disappear by the 12th day (provided that the elimination diet does not contain any idiopathic food sensitivities). They can also be reduced by taking buffered vitamin C and bread soda.

After three weeks on this diet you should have established a hypoallergenic baseline with the disappearance of all the symptoms. You can then start reintroducing suspect foods, one at a time while maintaining the low reactive elimination diet. Challenge with pure foods, not food mixtures or processed foods.

MONDAY

- **Breakfast:** Buckwheat porridge with rice milk and stewed pears.
- **Morning snack:** Raw cashews
- **Lunch:** Cold cooked rice and lentil salad with lettuce, mung bean sprouts, grated carrot, peas and shallots. Dress with sea salt, almond oil and sprinkle

with garlic.

- **Dinner:** Baked chicken with sweet potato, pumpkin and green beans.
- **Evening Snack:** Rock melon.

TUESDAY

- **Breakfast:** Puffed millet or rice bubbles with coconut milk and grated apple.
- **Morning Snack:** Rice cakes with hummus and celery sticks.
- **Lunch:** Vegetarian or salmon patties with salad (celery, carrot, bean shoots, shallots and lettuce).
- **Dinner:** Fresh fish (salmon, cod, whiting) with roast pumpkin and parsnips or green salad (lettuce, sprouts, shallots).
- **Evening Snack:** Pear (peeled). Drink purified water or herbal teas (chamomile, fennel, nettle).

WEDNESDAY

- **Breakfast:** Rock melon
- **Morning Snack**: Rice cakes with hummus.
- **Lunch:** Sliced turkey breast with steamed vegetables.
- **Dinner**: Gilled steak with sweet potatoes, carrots, green beans and turnips.
- **Evening Snack:** Avocado dip spread over buckwheat bread.

THURSDAY

- **Breakfast:** Buckwheat pancakes (mix buckwheat flour, sea salt, coconut milk, pear juice and cook with a little almond oil). Fill with banana and stewed pears).
- **Morning Snack:** Peeled red delicious apples.
- **Lunch:** Cooked scallops in lemon juice with salad of lettuce, bean sprouts, asparagus, grated carrot, celery and snow peas.

- **Dinner**: Roast lamb with roast vegetables (pumpkin, parsnip, carrots, sweet potato).

- **Evening Snack:** Mango and sago. Cook sago in rice milk for 10 minutes until thickened, add mango.

FRIDAY

- **Breakfast:** Rice bread toast with cashew paste and banana.
- **Morning Snack:** Carrot and celery sticks with hummus.
- **Lunch:** Lentil soup: stock (from steamed vegetables), sea salt, garlic, lentils, sweet potato, celery, carrot and leeks. Puree when cooked. Buckwheat bread.
- **Dinner:** Grill chicken breasts (sprinkled with sea salt, olive oil and garlic). Steamed vegetables: carrots, brussel sprouts, celery and cauliflower.
- **Evening Snack:** Macadamia nuts.

SATURDAY

- **Breakfast:** Rice bubbles with grated apple and coconut milk.
- **Morning Snack:** Peeled pear.
- **Lunch:** Sardines risotto with salad (lettuce, celery, mung bean sprouts, shallots).
- **Dinner:** Grilled salmon garnished with lemon juice and chives served with steamed carrots, cabbage and spinach.
- **Evening Snack:** Toasted rice cake with hummus.

SUNDAY

- **Breakfast:** Cook buckwheat kernels, millet and rice flakes in coconut milk until porridge consistency. Grate apple on top and sprinkle with cashews.

- **Morning Snack:** Rock melon
- **Lunch:** Cooked rice noodles with steamed vegetables: broccoli, bok choy, carrot, snow peas. Garnish with garlic in olive oil and sprinkle with chives.

- **Dinner:** Roast beef with cauliflower, sweet potato, pumpkin, peas and brussel sprouts.
- **Evening Snack:** Steamed peeled pear with cashew cream (blend raw cashews with a little water).

APPENDIX 5

EFFECTS OF COMMON FOODS ON THE BODY'S ACID/ALKALINE BALANCE

The ideal balance of acid-forming to alkaline-forming is 1:3. In other words, 75% of your dietary intake should be alkalising foods and 25% only to be derived from acid-forming foods. The simplest way to increase alkaline foods in your diet is to increase the amount of fresh fruit, vegetables and salads in the diet and to cut down on the less health-giving acid foods such as meat, sugar and dairy.

ACID-FORMING FOODS:

- All animal protein (beef, chicken, lamb, etc.
- All fried foods.
- All grains (wheat, rye, oats, corn, rice).
- All dairy products (milk, cheese, cream, etc.).
- All drugs and medicines.
- Alcohol.
- Artificial sweeteners.
- Beans and legumes.
- Coffee, tea and caffeinated products.
- Cocoa.
- Eggs.
- Fats and hydrogenated oils (animal and vegetable).
- Fruits (i.e. blueberries, cranberries, currants, prunes).
- Fish and shellfish.
- Flour products (i.e. breads, cakes, pastries).
- Junk and processed foods.
- Olives.
- Organ meats.
- Soft drinks.

- Sugar and products containing sugar.
- Tobacco and cigarettes.
- Vinegar, yeast and salad dressings.

ALKALINE–FORMING FOODS

- All vegetables.
- All sprouts (e.g. alfalfa, Mung beans).
- All leafy green salads.
- Avocados.
- Buckwheat, millet.
- Berries, most.
- Cold pressed oils (almond, olive, avocado, flax, sesame).
- Fruits (most including citrus fruits).
- Figs and dates.
- Garlic.
- Honey.
- Herbal teas.
- Juices, fresh fruit juice, green juices.
- Melons.
- Molasses, blackstrap.
- Herbs and spices.
- Mushrooms.
- Nuts: almonds Brazil.
- Natural sweeteners (Stevia).
- Potatoes and sweet potato.
- Super foods (spiralina, barley grass, wheat grass, chlorella).
- Sea salt.
- Sea veggies.
- Vinegar (apple cider and balsamic vinegar).
- Water, filtered.

References

1. Lipton, B. (2005). The Biology of Belief, Mountain of Love/Elite Books, California.
2. (WHO) Chapter 1 – Burden: Mortality, Morbidity and risk factors, www.who.int/nmh/publications/ncd_report_chapter1.pdf.
3. www.cdc.gov/nchs/nhanes/nhanes/nhanes.htm
4. www.wikipedia.org/wiki/healthy_diet
5. Holoford P. (2003) Depression: The Nutrition Connection: http://www.ingentaconnect.com/content/rmp/pcmh/2003/00000001/00000001/art00003
6. Centers for Disease Control and Prevention : National Diabetes Statistics Report, 2014.
7. Anne Underwood, Quieting a Body's Defences – Researchers are linking inflammation to an ever wider array of chronic illnesses, but treatments that block the inflammatory response can backfire. Newsweek, June 10, 2005.
8. Simopoulos AP. The importance of the ratio of omega-6/omega-3 essential fatty acids. Biomedicine and pharmacotherapy 2002; 56: 365-79.
9. Holman, RT, Geometrical and Positional Fatty Acid Isomers, EA Emkin and HJ Dutton, eds, 1979, American Oil Chemists Society, Champaign, 283-302; Science Newsletter, Feb. 1956; Schantz, EJ, et al, J Dairy Sci, 1940, 23: 181-89.
10. Enig, Mary G. PhD, Trans Fatty Acids in the Food Supply : A Comprehensive Report covering 60 years of Research, 2nd Edition, Enig Associates, Inc., Silver Spring, MD 1995,; Watkins, BA et al, Br Pouli Sci, Dec 1991, 32 (5) : 1109-1119.
11. Credit Suisse Research Institute, Sept 2013: Sugar Consumption at a Crossroads.
12. Lustig R. (2013) Fat Chance: Bloating the odds against Sugar Processed Food Obesity and Disease : New York, Hudson Street Press.
13. Trivedi, Bijal. "Food for Thought : Eat your way to Dementia". New Scientist

3rd Sept. 2012.

14. Warburg, O. On the Origin of Cancer Cells. Science 1956 Feb. 123 : 309-14.
15. Teng YT, Taylor GW et al. Periodontal health and Systemic Disorders. J Can Dent. Assoc. 2002; 67 : 188-92.
16. Hyman M. (2009). The Ultra Mind Solution. Scribner : Simon & Schuster N. Y. 10020.
17. Brown TP, et al 2006. Pesticides and Parkinson's Disease – Is there a link? Environmental Health Perspectives 114 (2) : 156-164.
18. Suk and Olden, 2005; Duncan D. 2006 The Pollution Within. National Geographic October 116 – 143.
19. http://medicalxpress.com/news/2014-08-mouth-bacteria-diet-supercomputers-reveal.html
20. Huebner FR et al. Demonstration of high opiad-like activity in isolated peptides from wheat gluten hydrolsates. Peptides. 1984 Nov. – Dec; 5 (6) : 1139=47.
21. Petersen AMW, Pederson BK. The anti-inflammatory effect of exercise. Journal of Applied Physiology: respiratory and exercise physiology 2005; 98 1154-62.
22. Lakka T.A. et al. Effect of exercise training on plasma levels of C-reactive protein in healthy adults: the HERITAGE Family Study. European heart journal 2005; 26: 2019-25.
23. Henriksen E.J. Exercise Effects of Muscle Insulin Signalling and Action Invited Review: Effect of acute exercise and exercise training on insulin resistance. J. Appl. Physiol. 93: 788-796, 2002.
24. How Does Exercise Affect our Mood? www.portfolio.mvm.ed.ac.uk
25. Neubauer O. et al. Recovery after an Ironman Triathlon: Sustained inflammatory responses and muscular stress. Dept. of Nut. Science University of Vienna 104 (3) 417-26 06/2008.
26. Over Training Syndrome Acute ME why exercise is dangerous for us. www.mecfsforums.com
27. Dr. Nibber : Could stress be affecting my thyroid gland? www.drnibber.com
28. Claire Viadro (May 2014) Sulphate, Sleep, Sunlight and Glyphosate. Nexus

Magazine Vol. 21, Number 5 Aug-Sept 2014.
29. http://m.sciencenewsline.com/news/2010111412000007
30. Mokdad AH, Ford ES, Bowman BA et al. Prevalence of obesity, diabetes, and obesity-related health risk factors, 2001. JAMA 2003 289: 76-9.
31. Greenberg AS, Obin MS, Obesity and the role of adipose tissue in inflammation and metabolism. The American Journal of Clinical Nutrition 2006. http://ajcn.nutrition.org/content/83/2/461S.full
32. Selvin E, Paynter NP et al. The Effect of Weight Loss on C-Reative Protein, A Systematic REview. JAMA Internal Medicine 2007 Vol 167, No. 1.
33. Hilden J.H. 1926 Toxemia Explained : The true interpretation of the cause of disease Denver, Colorado.
34. For more on the 4 R's go to: The Textbook of Functional Medicine at www.functionalmedicine.org
See article:
www.huffingtonpost.com/Jeffery_bland/chronic_illness_what_workb281228.html
35. Ehret A (1922) The Definitive Cure of Chronic Constipatiojn. Benedict Lust Publishers.
36. XUJ Gordon Jl. Inaugural article : honor ty smybionts. Proc Natt Acad Sci USA 100 10452-10459.
37. Blumenthal M, ed. The Complete German Commission E Monographs: Therapeutic Guide to Herbal Medicines. Austin TX: American Botanical Council; 1988.
38. Chappell LT & Stahl JP, J. Adv. Med. 1993; 6 : 139-60.
39. Barro WJ (1999) Lessons from the Miracle Doctors. www.jonbarron.org.
40. www.oilpulling.com
41. Ely. J.T.A. Heavy Metal Detox : Why Sweating May Protect the Kidneys. Will Dry Sauna prove the Safestand best method for most people? : from Well Mind Association Special Report – March 1994.
42. Examiner November 29, 2012: www.examiner.com/article/looking-to-sweat-new-infrared-sauna-studio-opens-delray-beach
43. Whelan HT et al, Effect of NASA light-emitting diode irradiation of wound

healing, J. Clin Laser Med Surg. 19 : 305-315, 2001.

44. Lockley S.W. – Division of Sleep Medicine http://sleep.med.harvard edu/people/faculty/163/steven+w+loc
45. www.senate.gov/reference/resources/pdf/modernmiraclemen.pdf
46. http://www.thewallachfiles.com/wallach.htm
47. Cheraskin E. et al, Establishing a suggested optimum nutrition allowance (SONA), 1994.
48. Bach E. The Twelve Healers: www.bachcentre.com/centre/download/healers.pdf
49. Book of Proverbs Ch. 23, verse 7.
50. Matthew: Ch. 15, verse 11.
51. Allen J. As a Man Thinketh : www.james-allen.in1woord.nl/text=as-a-man-thinketh
52. http://www.historybyzim.com/2011/11/all-roads-lead-to-rome/
53. Miguel Ruiz D (1997). The Four Agreements, Amber-Allen Publishing, San Rafael, California.
54. http://en.wikipedia.org/wiki/Desiderata
55. Leaves of Grass. http://en.wikipedia.org/wiki/Leaves_of_Grass
56. Becker RO, (1985). The Body Electric, William Morrow & Co. New York.
57. Glidden P (2014). The MD Emperor Has No Clothes, www.drglidden.com